Behavioral Classification System for Problem Behaviors in Schools

Ennio Cipani, PhD, is a licensed psychologist in California. He has published numerous articles, chapters, books, and software in the areas of child behavior management and behavioral consultation. His books include *Children and Autism: Stories of Hope and Triumph* (2011); *Punishment on Trial* (2004), which can be downloaded for free from the American Psychological Association Division 2 website (teachpsych.org/Resources/Documents/otrp/resources/cipani09 .pdf); and *Functional Behavioral Assessment, Diagnosis and Treatment: A Complete System for Education and Mental Health Settings* (Cipani & Schock, 2011). Dr. Cipani has been doing in-home and in-school behavioral consultation for children with problem behaviors since 1982. He has dealt with a variety of behavior problems and children with developmental and mental disabilities. He embodies a psychologist "who makes house calls" by conducting assessment and intervention activities in natural environments (i.e., homes and classrooms). He then provides on-the-spot training for direct-line people to engage in a parenting or teaching management repertoire that produces changes in undesirable child behavior.

There is a six module, author narrated, staff training video package detailing the Classification System that is freely available as a download to all school district personnel with bulk purchases of 15 or more copies. For more information about how to obtain the videos, please contact Ennio Cipani directly at EnnioC26@hotmail.com

Alessandra Cipani, MA, is currently a fourth-year school psychology doctoral student in the Graduate School of Education at the University of California, Riverside, where she received her MA in education with an emphasis on school psychology. After graduating with a BA from California State University San Marcos, she worked as a behavioral therapist, providing in-home applied behavior analysis interventions for toddlers, children, and adolescents. In addition to working in the field of applied behavior analysis, she is an active member of the National Association of School Psychologists (NASP). She plans to continue working and researching in both fields to provide comprehensive treatment plans that encompass home and school environments.

Behavioral Classification System for Problem Behaviors in Schools

A Diagnostic Manual

ENNIO CIPANI, PhD
ALESSANDRA CIPANI, MA

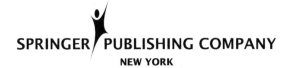

SPRINGER / PUBLISHING COMPANY
NEW YORK

Springer Publishing Company, LLC
11 West 42nd Street
New York, NY 10036
www.springerpub.com

Acquisitions Editor: Debra Riegert
Compositor: diacriTech

ISBN: 978-0-8261-7341-6
e-book ISBN: 978-0-8261-7342-3

Instructors Materials: Qualified instructors may request supplements by emailing textbook@springerpub.com:
Classification System PowerPoints: 978-0-8261-7345-4
Mistakes and Misconceptions PowerPoints: 978-0-8261-7347-8
Test Bank: 978-0-8261-7346-1

17 18 19 20 21 / 5 4 3 2 1

Library of Congress Cataloging-in-Publication Data
Names: Cipani, Ennio, author. | Cipani, Alessandra, author.
Title: Behavioral classification system for problem behaviors in schools : a
    diagnostic manual / Ennio Cipani and Alessandra Cipani.
Description: New York, NY : Springer Publishing Company, LLC, [2017] |
    Includes bibliographical references and index.
Identifiers: LCCN 2016054623| ISBN 9780826173416 | ISBN 9780826173423 (e-book)
Subjects: | MESH: Problem Behavior | Child | Applied Behavior
    Analysis—classification | Child Behavior Disorders—diagnosis | Adolescent
Classification: LCC RJ506.B44 | NLM WS 350.6 | DDC 618.92/89—dc23 LC record available at
https://lccn.loc.gov/2016054623

Printed in the United States of America by Gasch Printing.

FOR FACULTY INSTRUCTORS

If you are using this diagnostic manual for a course in school psychology, behavior analysis, or special education, instructor materials are available. These include test items for a final exam (along with a certificate of competence for inclusion in student portfolios) as well as PowerPoint slides (presentation material for about 3–6 hours of lecture to cover the diagnostic manual). To access these materials, send an e-mail to textbook@springerpub.com to establish that you are a faculty member teaching a course and have adopted the manual as required reading. You will then be given a password enabling you to download the materials.

You should also encourage your students to study the "Essential Terms to Know" at the beginning of the manual *as a prerequisite* to studying the actual diagnostic classification system. The underlying framework for this system may be new to many of your students. Acquiring the basic terms will help them make better sense of the material in this diagnostic manual.

CONTENTS

PREFACE

What Is It?

The Cipani Behavioral Classification System (BCS) is a pioneering function-based classification system for categorizing problem target behaviors in education and mental health settings. It was originally detailed in Cipani and Schock's *Functional Behavioral Assessment, Diagnosis and Treatment: A Complete System for Education and Mental Health Settings* (2007, 2011). This unique diagnostic classification system identifies four basic (operant) behavior functions and derives 13 different function-based categories within those four functions.

Using the Cipani BCS, functional treatment can be derived from the category selected (see Cipani & Schock, 2011). Personnel who conduct functional behavioral assessments (FBAs) can use this system of classification in their reports as a mechanism for conveying the function (environmental purpose) of problem behavior. It provides a stark contrast with symptom-based classification systems that categorize different topographies of behavior (as the unit for classifying behavioral phenomenon). Additionally, the numeric system allows for standardization translating a hypothesis about a behavior's function into a specific behavior–function category.

Why Is the Cipani BCS Needed?

Currently, hypotheses about the environmental function of problem behavior reported in FBAs are idiosyncratic, sometimes not even adhering to an environmental operant framework. For example, claiming the function of a particular student's problem behavior is manipulation[1] often appears in FBA reports. Yet, such a putative function does not even adhere to the theoretical principles of contextual environmental explanations. A common uniform set of possible functions, derived from environment–behavior relations, is needed.

It is also the case that use of "behavioral terminology" in the written report can mask poorly conceived assessment activities and capricious hypothesis selection. For example, in some FBAs, a well-sounding (but imprudent) hypothesis of "escape" is sometimes offered as the function for a target problem behavior. Such a contention may dupe a naïve person into trusting that a function has been meticulously identified (since it sounds behavioral?). Yet, such a hypothesis is troubling in its

---

1   All socially mediated operant behavior can be construed as being exhibited for the purpose of "manipulating" the social environment; that is, operant behavior "operates" on the environment.

ambiguity and connotes very little information (escape from what?). The only broad area that apparently has been ruled out are all access functions! In the Cipani BCS model, there are eight distinct escape functions. Consequently, use of this diagnostic system allows the written FBAs to become more precise with respect to the motivating condition (MC) that is "driving" the function.

In summary, the Cipani BCS[2] provides a standardized classification system for selecting a hypothesis about the function(s) of problem behavior for FBAs. Within four major categories, it presents 13 possible functions. Using this system, assessment activities are more expertly guided by a cognizance of a number of potential diverse functions, and assessment becomes an iterative process. The delineation of a diagnostic phase as an outcome of assessment activities, until now, has not been cogently presented in other FBA materials.

Clinical Utility

The principal utility of any classification system should be the straightforward path from diagnostic category to the subsequent selection of differential effective treatments. For example, an intervention for a problem maintained by escape from instruction due to task difficulty will be markedly different than an intervention derived for a problem maintained by adult/staff attention. Therefore, two separate and distinct interventions plans should follow.

Suppose a particular child is verbally aggressive under both sets of conditions (i.e., task difficulty and absence of attention). Staff would intervene differentially, depending on which condition is in effect (i.e., escape from difficult task function or attention function). This is an important point and one that is often overlooked in practice. The use of this function-based classification system guides such a derivation of differing intervention plans as a result of classifying function.[3]

If function does not determine differential interventions, one would simply select an intervention based on some other characteristic; for example, behavioral interventions that are deemed appropriate

---

2   Questions, comments, or feedback about the utility of this manual—as well as requests for information about webinar training or on-demand narrations for teachers and other school personnel that supplements this manual—can be directed to Ennio Cipani at ennioc26@hotmail .com, using "diagnostic manual comment" in the subject line.

3   For a complete delineation of functional treatment for each of the four major categories, the reader is enjoined to examine Chapter 4 of Cipani & Schock (2011). In particular, tolerance training for escape functions should be carefully examined for its application to problems involving the student's inability to handle aversive events such as instructional tasks (that are within his or her capability).

for children with attention deficit hyperactivity disorder (ADHD). Unfortunately, disorders derived from prior editions or the current fifth edition of the *Diagnostic and Statistical Manual of Mental Disorders (DSM;* American Psychiatric Association, 2013*)* classification system (or in the case of the education codes, disability categories) have not been shown to have any behavioral treatment selection utility. One does not prescribe *time-out* because such a procedure only works with ADHD children, and concurrently has been found to be not effective with other childhood mental disorders! Rather, time-out should be prescribed when such a procedure affects the existing behavior–environment relations, irrespective of the putative *DSM* diagnosis. Hence, knowing that a particular child has been diagnosed with ADHD is of little benefit in determining how to treat noncompliance in that particular child. In contrast, functionally derived interventions have been proven over the past several decades to yield effective treatment of problem behavior (see issues of major journals, such as the *Journal of Applied Behavior Analysis*, over the past several decades for such studies; also see reviews by Beavers, Iwata, & Lerman, 2013; Hanley, Iwata, & McCord, 2003).

An additional corollary of a functional approach to the classification of problem behavior is that problem behaviors occurring at an unacceptable rate (or dangerous forms) are not viewed as symptomatic of a disorder (Cipani, 2014). Rather such behaviors are understood as functional given their contextual basis. (As an example of such a contextual approach, go to https://youtu.be/qtgokxRcU_w for a presentation on a behavior–analytic formulation of childhood aggression, narrated by Ennio Cipani.

Accuracy of Category Selection

The selection of a hypothesized function is derived from the assessment data that is collected regarding behavior and environmental variables. Hence, the accuracy of a particular selected diagnostic classification is dependent on the accuracy and type of assessment evidence obtained for any particular case. The types of descriptive and experimental assessment methods that can yield a behavior's function are delineated in Cipani and Schock (2011). It is not the objective of this manual to elucidate all such methods, but it is recommended that the reader consult this reference for a comprehensive view of these methods.

In this diagnostic manual, an in-vivo assessment method that establishes the hypothesized MC termed *trigger analysis* (Cipani & Schock, 2011; Rolider & Axelrod, 2000) is offered for most classification categories. This allows the user to collect experimental evidence regarding a specific hypothesis selected. This method involves the presentation of the putative MC, or "trigger," conducted "in vivo" with personnel endemic to the natural context. Given the measure is obtained in the natural setting, it should yield valid data on actual behavior–environment relations. For most of the classification categories, a divergent validity test (using an alternate hypothesis test) is also provided. It is the decision of the individual user of this classification system to determine if one or both tests are warranted for any particular case. For additional material on using the trigger analysis with behavioral description to examine qualitative (i.e., the behavioral descriptions in the middle column), as well as quantitative information, please see Chapter 2 in Cipani and Schock (2011).

The Cipani BCS is theoretically sound as it is procured from the four major functions of operant behavior (following nomenclature used in Cipani & Schock, 2007, 2011, and preceded by Cipani, 1990, 1994): (a) Socially Mediated Access (SMA), (b) Direct Access (DA), (c) Socially Mediated Escape (SME), and (d) Direct Escape (DE). Hence, such is content-valid given the extensive and longitudinal history of work and research in behavior analysis experimentally demonstrating functional relationships between behavior and its environmental outcome.[4]

From these four major categories of behavioral function, the Cipani BCS derives 13 subcategories or specific functions under these primary generic functions. Each of the classifications under a given major category shares all the characteristics of that category, except for the specific stimuli that are involved in the particular function. For example, the major category of SMA involves the following: under an MC involving a state of deprivation with respect to an item/activity/event, the problem target behavior(s) is effective in producing the desired event relative to other behaviors. This characteristic is shared among all three categories within the SMA. The distinction between these three categories (2.1, 2.2, and 2.3) is the type of item or activity that is in a deprived state for that person. In the case of SMA 2.1, it is the absence of adult/staff attention. In the case of SMA 2.2, it is the absence of peer attention. In the case of SMA 2.3, it is the absence of a specific tangible item, activity, or event. Subsequently, the environmental outcome of the functional behavior also differs as a result of these slight differences in the MC.

The other three major categories of functions have the same relationship to the classifications within their domain. If the characteristics of each major category serve as an operational definition, then the classifications derived from each, which follow the same operational definitions, are also content valid.

---

4   See these research reviews of functional analysis methodology across a wide spectrum of problem behaviors: Beavers et al. (2013); Hanley et al. (2003).

THE CIPANI BEHAVIORAL CLASSIFICATION SYSTEM

CATEGORIES

- Direct Access (DA 1.0) Functions
  - DA 1.1: Immediate Sensory Stimuli
  - DA 1.2: Tangible Reinforcers
- Socially Mediated Access (SMA 2.0) Functions
  - SMA 2.1: Adult/Staff Attention
  - SMA 2.2: Peer Attention
  - SMA 2.3: Tangible Reinforcers
- Direct Escape (DE 3.0) Functions
  - DE 3.1: Unpleasant Social Situations
  - DE 3.2: Lengthy Tasks, Chores, or Assignments
  - DE 3.3: Difficult Tasks, Chores, or Assignments
  - DE 3.4: Aversive Physical Stimuli or Event
- Socially Mediated Escape (SME 4.0) Functions
  - SME 4.1: Unpleasant Social Situations
  - SME 4.2: Lengthy Tasks, Chores, or Assignments
  - SME 4.3: Difficult Tasks, Chores, or Assignments
  - SME 4.4: Aversive Physical Stimuli or Event

ESSENTIAL TERMS TO KNOW

- **Access function[1]:** Behavior produces a desired item or event under a relative state of deprivation that makes such a behavior functional under that antecedent context. The environmental outcome of the behavior is to "access/obtain" an item, activity, or event.

- **Escape function[2]:** Behavior terminates (or postpones advent of) an item or event under a relative state of aversion that makes such a behavior functional under that antecedent context. The environmental outcome of the behavior is to "escape or avoid" an impending or presented item, activity, or event.

- **Socially mediated function:** Reinforcer (i.e., desired outcome) is produced through the behavior of another person. This can occur for both access and escape functions.

- **Direct function[3]:** Reinforcer (i.e., desired outcome) is produced through the behavior's explicit contact with the physical environment. This can occur for both access and escape functions.

- **Motivating condition[4] (MC) for access functions:** An absence of the desired item, activity, or event (including sensations such as auditory, visual, etc.) *at that point in time* creates a *sufficient* state of deprivation that (a) such items, activities, or events become more valued (compared to other events or escape from aversive events) and (b) behaviors that produce such become more probable at that point in time (Cipani & Schock, 2011; Michael, 1993, 2007). The MC (i.e., state of deprivation) is the *driving force* behind an operable function.

- **MC[5] for escape functions:** The presence (or impending presentation) of an aversive (nonpreferred) item, activity, or event for the individual *at that point in time* creates a *sufficient* state of aversion that (a) termination/removal of the ongoing aversive stimulus item, activity, or event becomes more valued (compared to other present or impending aversive events or access to desired items/activities) and (b) behaviors that are effective in terminating (or avoiding) such become more

---

1   Termed a *positive reinforcement function* in behavior analysis literature.
2   Termed a *negative reinforcement function* in behavior analysis literature.
3   Termed *automatic reinforcement* in behavior analysis literature.
4   Termed an *establishing operation* (EO) in behavior analysis literature (antecedent event to behavior).
5   Termed an *EO* in behavior analysis literature (antecedent event to behavior).

probable at that point in time (Cipani & Schock, 2011; Michael, 1993, 2007). The MC (i.e., state of aversion) is the *driving force* behind an operable function.

- **Behavioral function:** A behavioral function is a reliable temporally proximate behavior[6]–environment relationship that produces an outcome that abolishes or abates the relevant MC at that point in time. A common mistake is the assumption that the initial socially mediated event that occurs after the behavior dictates the function. While there are many social and physical environmental consequences of any behavior, the function is dictated by the consequent event that abolishes or abates the given MC at that time ("driving force"). For socially mediated functions, adult attention and proximity follow the functional behavior, but such may not be the "reason" for the functional behavior. Such attention is endemic to events that are socially mediated. Hence, their occurrence just correlates with the true function, but does not act in a causal manner.

- **Trigger analysis** (Cipani & Schock, 2011; Rolider & Axelrod, 2000): An experimental in vivo assessment methodology that involves procedures that contrive a putative MC at a point in time to experimentally determine if such an antecedent condition is functionally related to the target problem behavior. This is done by conducting such a test trial when the target behavior is not occurring.

  This method is far superior to the more commonly used A-B-C charts to detect function. The latter often miss the antecedent MC for access functions, which is the absence of some event or item. Further, simply identifying the initial consequent action of an adult does not reveal that such is the "true" function of that behavior. Many events occur subsequent to a problem behavior. *A problem behavior's function is revealed only when the MC at that point in time is determined.* This axiom of an operant behavioral function is entrenched in this diagnostic manual. Each separate classification category is defined by its unique MC and behavior–environment mechanism for achieving the designated function.

---

6   Such a definition of behavior should actually be a class of behaviors that act in a similar fashion on the environment; that is, produce the designated function under a given MC.

SECTION I: DIAGNOSTIC MANUAL

DIRECT ACCESS (DA 1.0) FUNCTIONS

- DA 1.1: Immediate Sensory Stimuli
- DA 1.2: Tangible Reinforcers

GENERAL DESCRIPTION

Direct access (DA) functions involve behavior that effectively and efficiently *directly* produces a desired item or event (or specific sensation, auditory, visual, kinesthetic, etc.). The event or item in the physical environment is contacted and obtained directly by the individual's behavior. Such an item or activity is sufficiently deprived at that particular point in time to be of value (in relation to other possible MCs); hence, an MC exists for such items/events. The DA functions contrast with the other type of access functions: socially mediated access (SMA), in which the behavior produces the desired item or event by inducing another person to provide it (Table 1.1).

Table 1.1: Examples of DA functions

MC	Behavior	Function of behavior
Desires potato chips	Goes to cupboard and retrieves item	Gets potato chips
Desires specific auditory sensation, in shower area	Sings in shower	Sound produced (which is reinforcing at that time)
Desires to play on swing	Runs out of classroom and jumps on swing, no one impedes such	Gets to swing unencumbered for 15 minutes (until sated for this activity, then comes back into classroom)

The three examples in Table 1.1 all illustrate that the end result of the behavior is the immediate direct contact with the desired item or event. In the first example, the chain of behaviors leads to consumption of the desired item. In example two, the singing produced a desired auditory sensation. In the last example, the chain of behaviors results in engagement in the desired activity.

Such behaviors are often more efficient than behaviors that attempt to achieve their desired effect through social mediation. However, when the ability to contact the desired event or item *directly* is impeded (by school staff, other adults, etc.), such behaviors become less probable. This obstruction of behaviors that produce DA behaviors can result in the genesis and development of problem behaviors that achieve their effect by acting on the social environment (see next major category, SMA).

- Under Motivating Conditions (MC), problem target behavior(s) is effective in *directly* (without social mediation) producing the sensory event desired. Such sensory effects produced immediately from such behaviors can include visual, auditory, gustatory, tactile, and olfactory stimuli.

MC for DA 1.1

An absence of the desired sensation *at that point in time* creates a *sufficient* state of deprivation with respect to the sensation that (a) such become more valued (compared to other events or escape from aversive events) and (b) such a stereotypic display produces such a desired sensation immediately and for the length of time it occurs.

Diagnostic Criteria
1. Presence of MC for DA 1.1.
2. The form of the stereotypic behavior is more effective/efficient than other behaviors at immediately producing the desired sensory event under the MC.

All of the examples in Table 1.2 exhibit a behavior that immediately produces the desired sensation, whether it is auditory, kinesthetic, or other. Many ritualistic behaviors can be maintained by their sensory effects, or the effects on the physical environment; for example, arranging chairs every day in a specific fashion (usually with respect to very inconspicuous aspects of each chair).

Experimental verification: Since the MC for this category is a private event, with awareness only to the individual desiring such, a trigger analysis is not plausible. However, Querim et al. (2013) found that in many cases, just three or four, 5-minute sessions involving an "alone or no interaction" condition allow one to draw a conclusion regarding the plausibility of this category as the operative function. Simply allow the individual to be alone with no interaction and

---

7   In studying this diagnostic manual for the first time, it would be wise to review all the other functions first that have great commonality. This classification, DA 1.1: Immediate Sensory Stimuli, is a unique function in the nature of the MC and the outcome of behavior (both are unobservable but inferred). My recommendation is that it is easier to understand examples that have shared characteristics first and then study and learn of a unique case example (e.g., DA 1.1).

record the rate of the target problem behavior. Conceivably, to set up a state of deprivation with respect to the sensory event, one could have a presession where access to the sensory event is removed or impeded. Then immediately provide unlimited access in the alone condition (of course for school settings, supervision should be present).

Table 1.2: Examples of sensory stimuli function

MC	Behavior	Result on desired outcome	Future likelihood of behavior (under MC)
1:35 p.m. Desires a specific auditory sensory event	1:35 p.m. Puts hand to ear cupped and hums into hand	Produces auditory stimulus	Form of self-stimulatory behavior becomes more refined and proficient
12:05 p.m. Desires a kinesthetic sensory event	12:05 p.m. Rocks back and forth	Produces movement and unique kinesthetic sensation	Such a form will occur because of the immediate sensation produced
8:07 a.m. Desires a specific visual sensory event	8:07 a.m. Throws mud against wall and sees it go *splat*	Throwing mud produces unique visual result	Throwing mud will occur when the mud is available (after a rain)[8]

---

8   One may not see the behavior when only dirt is on the ground, since the visual effect of dirt hitting the wall is not quite the same.

DA 1.2: TANGIBLE REINFORCERS

▪ Under MCs, problem target behavior(s) is effective in *directly* (without social mediation) producing the desired item, activity, or event (i.e., tangible reinforcer). Such items can include food, drink, particular food or drink, individual or group activities such as games, sports, dances, social conversation and interaction, phone use, computer use, weekend outings, time with friends, and so on. Realize that tangible reinforcers (desired items or events) can often be idiosyncratic with respect to each individual. For example, reading a nonfiction book, at certain times is a highly desired activity for some people, while for other people it constitutes an undesirable activity (i.e., sets up avoidance or escape conditions).

MC for DA 1.2
An absence of the desired item, activity, or event for the individual *at that point in time* creates a *sufficient* state of deprivation with respect to the item, activity, or event that (a) such become more valued (compared to other events or escape from aversive events) and (b) DA behaviors that produce such become more probable at that point in time (given they are not impeded or encumbered).

Diagnostic Criteria
1. Presence of MC for DA 1.2.
2. Target problem behavior(s) is more effective/efficient than other behaviors at directly contacting/producing the tangible reinforcer under the MC, far greater reliable relation between target behavior and tangible reinforcer (as opposed to the relation of other behaviors and their ability to access that item, event, or activity; Table 1.3).

Table 1.3: Example 1 of tangible reinforcer function

MC	DA behavior	Result on desired outcome	Future likelihood of behavior (under MC)
11:25 a.m. Wants to doodle on paper (instead of doing seat work)	11:25 a.m. Gets a blank paper, puts it under math assignment, and covertly draws Star Wars characters on paper	Spends time doodling and drawing Star Wars characters	If sufficiently stealthy, such doodling likely when staff are occupied and unable to detect off-task behavior

Explanation: When this student is given seatwork at 11:25 a.m., his preference at that time is to engage in a drawing task involving Star Wars characters. Due to the surreptitious nature of this behavior, the student's doodling and drawing activity go undetected. Certainly less clandestine attempts will likely result in the drawing activity being impeded, so the individual learns to become stealthier to avoid detection. Over time, it becomes more probable, given these conditions (Table 1.4).

Table 1.4: Example 2 of tangible reinforcer function

MC	Behavior	Result on desired outcome	Future likelihood of behavior (under MC)
1:35 p.m. Wants to play with toys in backpack	1:35 p.m. Opens up backpack and gets toys out	Gets to play with toys	More likely (if unencumbered by teaching staff)

Explanation: Under the MC of desiring a play activity with toys at 1:35 p.m., the child engages in a chain of behaviors that result in access to toys in her backpack. If such behavior is left unimpeded, access is both direct and efficient/effective. However, if staff hinder and interrupt such play in subsequent occurrences, this form of access may be replaced with other behaviors that may become more successful (such often takes the form of SMA functions).

Trigger Analysis Procedures

- Set a ceiling limit for the duration of the trial; for example, 5 minutes, 8 minutes, and so on. (If the initial time ceiling is insufficient, increase it in subsequent trials and use that data only; delete prior data from previous ceiling.)
- Always obtain written consent to perform these tests as part of the assessment process for problem behaviors.
- If a dangerous behavior (to self, property, or others) is the target problem, then select a precursor behavior, upon which the desired item or activity will be immediately provided contingently.
- This assessment method for DA 1.2 is similar to that deployed for SMA 2.3: Tangible Reinforcer, except the target behavior is a DA form, for example, getting the item (activity or event) oneself without permission.
- To induce a state of deprivation with respect to the tangible item or activity, after providing the item/activity for a short period of time (e.g., a few minutes), remove the item/activity from the student. At the same time, contrive the environment so as to make it available to the individual upon the chain of DA (target) behaviors. For example, place the item in view and within reach of the student. Then leave the immediate area to allow the DA behavior to be successful in retrieving the item. If the desired item is consumable, in order to affect the trigger analysis, do the following. Provide just a small amount of the food item (to set up the desire for more), and then leave the remaining food item in an area that is easily accessible to the individual.
- When the target behavior occurs, provide the desired item or event at that time. The trial ends at that point.
- Record a plus if the target behavior (or precursor behavior) occurs within the time limit (i.e., before the ceiling) or a minus if it did not.
- Provide a minimum (over several days) of five trials or until a pattern emerges, that is, most occurrences or nonoccurrences.

Divergent Validity: *See* **Adult/Staff Attention: Trigger Analysis**

Conduct the attention trigger analysis as a control (contrast) condition for the above assessment of tangible reinforcer function.

If the data collected in this divergent validity test show a low or zero level of target behavior (or precursor if that was selected for analysis aforementioned), divergent validity is established. One can put greater confidence in the selection of the DA 1.2 function. If the rate of the target behavior is high under this divergent validity test, then a DA 1.2 seems unlikely. Rather, an SMA 2.1: Adult/Staff Attention should be entertained. Further anecdotal evidence during the divergent validity test for an SMA 2.1 classification being operative would be the following observation: The target behavior stops immediately or shortly after adult attention is given.

SOCIALLY MEDIATED ACCESS (SMA 2.0) FUNCTIONS

- SMA 2.1: Adult/Staff Attention
- SMA 2.2: Peer Attention
- SMA 2.3: Tangible Reinforcers

GENERAL DESCRIPTION

SMA functions involve behavior that effectively and efficiently produces a desired item or event (through someone's acting on such behavior). Such an item or activity is sufficiently deprived at that particular point in time to be of value (relative to other possible motivating conditions [MCs]); hence, an MC exists for such items/events. All three examples in Table 1.5, despite having different behavioral topographies, have the same function, that is, getting potato chips from someone, under a given MC.

Table 1.5: Examples of SMA functions

MC	Behavior	Function of behavior
Desires potato chips	Asks for potato chips	Gets item
Desires potato chips	Makes rude request, "Give me the $##%% chips!"	Gets item
Desires potato chips	Hits self	Gets item

Under MCs, problem target behavior(s) is effective in producing desired adult/staff attention relative to other behaviors. Such adult/staff attention can be in the form of vocal comments and interaction, as well as nonvocal behaviors including eye contact, gestures, physical contact, and/or close proximity.

MC for SMA 2.1

An absence of adult/staff attention for the individual *at that point in time* creates a *sufficient* state of deprivation with respect to adult/staff attention that (a) adult/staff attention becomes more valued (compared to other events or escape from aversive events) and (b) behaviors that produce such attention become more probable at that point in time.

Diagnostic Criteria

1. Presence of MC for SMA 2.1.
2. Target problem behavior(s) is more effective/efficient than other behaviors at producing attention under the MC; far greater reliable relation between target behavior and attention (as opposed to the relation of other behaviors and their ability to access adult/staff attention).
3. Presence of person(s) who has a history of producing attention under the specific MC for target problem behaviors (person is discriminative for providing attention for such behaviors). See Table 1.6 for an analysis of an adult/staff attention function.
4. **Special note**: Adult attention and close proximity will always be consequent to the behavior for functions that are socially mediated (e.g., SMA and socially mediated escape [SME] functions). The desired result is achieved only via social (human) mediation. Hence, an adult's presence/attention is endemic to such functions. But do not equate such a proximal temporal relationship with the actual function in all these circumstances. If the value of attention at that point in time relative to the other operable MCs is inferior, the function of the behavior is not simply adult attention; rather it is the access to a tangible reinforcer (or for SME functions, the termination of the aversive state). Therefore, a diagnosis of SME 2.1: Adult Attention is not correct when other MCs exert more of an effect on the value of reinforcers other than adult/staff attention. The function that is

---

9   Be aware that access to peer attention for behavior often occurs when the teacher publicly attends to behavior.

"driving force" in these circumstances is the category whose MC is producing the greatest influence at that point in time.

Table 1.6: Example 1 of adult/staff attention function

MC	Behavior	Result on desired outcome	Future likelihood of behavior (under MC)
9:30 a.m. Desires teacher attention	9:30 a.m. Holds up hand to get teacher attention (about 30 in.)	Told to wait	Less likely
	9:40 a.m. Says, "I really need help, please!"	Ignored	Less likely
Still desires teacher attention (possibly even more so!)	9:45 a.m. "Can I get some help here, for crying out loud?" (in a rude manner)	Teacher comes over. "Can you ask nicely next time? Okay, what do you want?"	Calling out in a rude fashion becomes more likely than other ineffective behaviors

Explanation: Under the MC of desiring teacher attention, the rude request, "Can I get some help here?" at 9:45 a.m. produces the desired event: teacher attention (see last row). Other behaviors, such as raising hand or asking nicely (see first two rows), occurred prior to the target problem behavior and did not result in the teacher coming over to help. Hence, one can see that such behaviors are not functional under the MC (and hence will become less probable). Attention would appear to be more available for a more undesirable form of request. If this scenario plays out again and again over time, such rude requests become very likely when the desire for attention is great (Table 1.7).

Table 1.7: Example 2 of adult/staff attention function

MC	Behavior	Result on desired outcome	Future likelihood of behavior (under MC)
11:30 a.m. Teacher is playing with a fellow student during recess; desires teacher attention (currently unavailable)	11:30 a.m. "Ms. Jones, look at what I am doing."	Teacher continues playing with other child	Less likely
	11:43 a.m. Starts crying in a whimper	Ignored, continues with other child	Less likely
	11:45 a.m. Crying continues but louder and audible to all	Teacher comes over. "Billy what is the matter? Let's play with this," and engages with child	Crying at a certain decibel level becomes more probable, whimpering softly is less likely

Explanation: Under the motivating condition of desiring adult/staff attention, at 11:30 a.m. the child makes an appropriate request for the teacher to attend to him, but it is not effective in getting the teacher to leave the current activity and come over to the child. The same result (or lack thereof) occurs for soft crying and whimpering a short time later. But louder crying at 11:45 a.m. is effective in getting the teacher to leave the one child and come over to Billy. In the future, when the teacher is with someone else and Billy wants her attention, he will resort (much sooner) to loud crying, as it is more effective (functional) than other behaviors.

Trigger Analysis Procedures

- Set a ceiling limit for the duration of the trial (e.g., 5 minutes, 8 minutes; if the initial time ceiling is insufficient, increase it in subsequent trials and use that data only; delete prior data from previous ceiling).
- Always obtain written consent to perform these tests as part of the assessment process for problem behaviors.

- If a dangerous behavior (to self, property, or others) is the target problem, then select a precursor behavior, upon which attention will be immediately provided contingently.
- To induce a state of deprivation with respect to attention, after providing attention for a short period of time (e.g., a few minutes), remove attention by leaving the target individual and going over to another individual and providing attention to him or her.
- When the target behavior occurs, provide attention for a period of time; the trial ends at that point.
- Record a plus, if the target behavior (or precursor behavior) occurs within the time limit (i.e., before the ceiling) or a minus if it did not.
- Provide a minimum (over several days) of five trials or until a pattern emerges (i.e., most occurrences or nonoccurrences).

Divergent validity test—none (but it is recommended that another category of function be considered first unless there is considerable anecdotal evidence pointing to attention as the maintaining contingency). In school settings, I have found (Ennio Cipani) that other functions (e.g., 2.3, 4.2, or 4.3) are more often the operable function.

SMA 2.2: PEER ATTENTION

Under MCs, problem target behavior(s) is effective in producing desired peer attention relative to other behaviors. Such peer attention can be in the form of vocal comments and interaction, as well as nonvocal behaviors including eye contact, gestures, physical contact, and/or close association such as friendship, continued affiliation with individual as part of a group.

MC for SMA 2.2

An absence of desired peer attention for the individual *at that point in time* creates a *sufficient* state of deprivation with respect to peer attention that (a) a specific peer's or group's attention becomes more valued (compared to other events or escape from aversive events) and (b) behaviors that produce such peer attention become more probable at that point in time.

Diagnostic Criteria

1. Presence of MC for SMA 2.2.
2. Target problem behavior(s) is more effective/efficient than other behaviors at producing peer attention under the MC; far greater reliable relation between target behavior and attention (as opposed to the relation of other behaviors and their ability to access adult/staff attention).
3. Presence of peer(s) who has a history of producing attention under the specific MC for target problem behaviors (peers are discriminative for providing attention for such behaviors; Table 1.8).

Table 1.8: Example 1 of peer attention function

MC	Behavior	Result on desired outcome-peer's attention	Future likelihood of behavior (under MC)
9:30 a.m. Desires peer attention (a possible love interest sits next to individual)	9:32 a.m. "I am hungry!"	Not effective	
	9:37 a.m. Opens up textbook	Ignored	
Still desires peer attention	9:38 a.m. "This class %$@@"	Person who is target of affections smiles and agrees	Such derogatory comments more likely

Explanation: Under the MC of desiring a specific peer's attention, the first comment was ineffective (not dramatic enough). Also, opening up the textbook to the assignment does not result in the desired peer attention.[10] However, the caustic comment about the class does produce such attention. Hence, such comments will occur more frequently if they continue to recruit desired attention from a peer(s) (Table 1.9).

---

10   As a side comment, it is the unfortunate case that many desirable behaviors at older grade levels are ineffective in acquiring peer attention, unless a group contingency is in place.

Table 1.9: Example 2 of peer attention function

MC	Behavior	Result on desired outcome	Future likelihood of behavior (under MC)
10:00 a.m. Peer attention desired. Such becomes available with teacher's request, "Bob can you go sit down?"	10:00 a.m. "I don't want to sit down. You sit down if you like it so much!"	Peers observe such an interaction	Very likely (when it recruits attention and future "respect" from classmates

Explanation: Under the MC of a request from the teacher, this student makes a derogatory comment. Such not only accesses peer attention at that time, but may also produce a level of "respect" among other students (e.g., "Boy, Bob is pretty tough!"). Such derogatory comments become more common when sufficient consequences for such behaviors are either (a) not applied or (b) are unavailable due to other constraints (e.g., policy on such consequences).

Trigger Analysis Procedures

Such an assessment is not viable given the nature of peer attention. See in situ hypothesis testing (Cipani & Schock, 2011, Chapter 2) for a potentially useful test.

Divergent Validity: *See* Adult/Staff Attention: Trigger Analysis

Conduct the attention trigger analysis to rule out adult attention as a possible explanation of behavior.

If the data collected in this divergent validity test show a low or zero level of target behavior (or precursor if that was selected for analysis aforementioned), divergent validity is established. One can put greater confidence in the selection of the SMA 2.2 function. If the rate of the target behavior is high under this divergent validity test, then an SMA 2.2 seems unlikely. Rather, an SMA 2.1: Adult/Staff Attention should be entertained. Further anecdotal evidence during the divergent validity test for an SMA 2.1 classification being operative would be the following observation: The target behavior stops immediately or shortly after adult attention is given.

Under MCs, problem target behavior(s) is effective in producing desired item, activity, or event (i.e., tangible reinforcer) by the action of someone else, (i.e., social mediation). Such items can include food, drink, particular food or drink, individual or group activities such as games, sports, dances, social conversation and interaction, phone use, computer use, weekend outings, or time with friends. Realize that tangible reinforcers (desired items/events) can often be idiosyncratic with respect to each individual. For example, reading a nonfiction book, at certain times is a highly desired activity for some people, while for other people it constitutes an undesirable activity (i.e., sets up avoidance or escape conditions).

MC for SMA 2.3

An absence of the desired item, activity, or event for the individual *at that point in time* creates a *sufficient* state of deprivation with respect to the item, activity, or event that (a) such become more valued (compared to other events or escape from aversive events) and (b) behaviors that produce such become more probable at that point in time.

Diagnostic Criteria

1. Presence of MC for SMA 2.3.
2. Target problem behavior(s) is more effective/efficient than other behaviors at producing the tangible reinforcer under the MC; far greater reliable relation between target behavior and tangible reinforcer (as opposed to the relation of other behaviors and their ability to access that item, event, or activity).
3. Presence of person(s) who has a history of producing the tangible reinforcer under the specific MC for target problem behaviors (person is discriminative for providing desired item/activity for such behaviors; Tables 1.10 and 1.11).

Table 1.10: Example 1 of tangible reinforcer function

MC	Behavior	Result on desired outcome	Future likelihood of behavior (under MC)
12:30 p.m. Desires a special cookie	12:30 p.m. "Can I have that cookie?"	Does not get cookie, told to wait until tomorrow	
12:42 p.m.	Twelve minutes elapse, then asks again	Same as above	
	12:43 p.m. Starts whimpering	Ignored, no cookie	
	12:46 p.m. Falls to the floor and screams for several minutes	Gets cookie after lengthy tantrum (told to get up and then given cookie)	Tantrum behaviors become more likely in the future under MC

Explanation: Under the MC of wanting a special cookie, the child's appropriate request is ineffective (see first entry). After waiting for 12 minutes, a second request also goes unmet. However, a lengthy tantrum accompanied by falling to the floor was the "key" to getting this particular adult to provide the desired cookie. One should conclude that waiting for tomorrow is only operative if the request does not involve falling to the floor and creating a scene!

Table 1.11: Example 2 of tangible reinforcer function

MC	Behavior	Result on desired outcome	Future likelihood of behavior (under MC)
2:15 p.m. Desires time on the computer	2:15 p.m. Asks the teacher, "Can I get on the computer?"	Ineffective, told, "You will have to wait until 3 p.m.!"	
	2:35 p.m. Waited for 20 minutes	Ignored, no computer	
	2: 36 p.m. Asks again	Told that he needs to wait a little bit longer	
	2:38 p.m. Begins teasing other students at 2:36 until 2:38 p.m.	Put on computer to redirect his "energies"	Teasing becomes more likely at this time

Explanation: Under the MC of desiring time on the computer at 11:30 a.m., the child makes two requests that fall on an unreceptive staff person. Also note that the child did manage to wait for 20 minutes, but such desirable behavior was not effective at that level in producing computer access (second entry). However, bothering other students for several minutes was sufficient to get the staff person to put the child on the computer to circumvent further teasing to other students. Such an "undesirable demand form" is the way to go in this circumstance, and the adult will become discriminative for the specific reinforcement of such behavior.

Trigger Analysis Procedures

- Set a ceiling limit for the duration of the trial (e.g., 5 minutes, 8 minutes; if the initial ceiling is insufficient, increase it in subsequent trials and use that data only; delete prior data from previous ceiling).
- Always obtain written consent to perform these tests as part of the assessment process for problem behaviors.
- If a dangerous behavior (to self, property, or others) is the target problem, then select a precursor behavior, upon which desired tangible reinforcer will be immediately provided contingently.

- To induce a state of deprivation with respect to the tangible item or activity, after providing the item (small amount) or activity (for a short period of time; e.g., a few minutes), remove/withdraw the activity or make the remaining amount of the item unavailable. If the tangible item is consumable, provide only a small amount of the food item. Then leave the area with the remaining amount of food to contrive the child's desire for more.
- When the target behavior occurs, provide the desired tangible reinforcer for a period of time; the trial ends at that point.
- Record a plus if the target behavior (or precursor behavior) occurs within the time limit (i.e., before the ceiling) or a minus if it did not.
- Provide a minimum (over several days) of five trials or until a pattern emerges (i.e., most occurrences or nonoccurrences).

Divergent Validity: *See* adult/staff attention: trigger analysis
Conduct the attention trigger analysis as a control (contrast) condition for the above assessment of tangible reinforcer function. Since the provision of a tangible reinforcer involves another person providing it, attention/proximity are inherently involved; therefore, one should test for attention only (without any tangible item/activity). Such a contrast allows one to separate out the contaminating effects of attention as an inherent component in all socially mediated functions.

If the data collected in this divergent validity test show a low or zero level of target behavior (or precursor if that was selected for analysis aforementioned), divergent validity is established. One can put greater confidence in the selection of the SMA 2.3 function. If rates of behavior are somewhat comparable between these two types of the tests (i.e., target behavior almost or just as likely to occur with attention as the only event following it), then one cannot unambiguously state that SMA 2.3 selection of function is unequivocal. This would be also evident in the divergent validity test. One would observe anecdotally that when attention is provided for the target behavior, it stops immediately or shortly after.

DIRECT ESCAPE (DE 3.0) FUNCTIONS

- **DE 3.1: Unpleasant Social Situations**
- **DE 3.2: Lengthy Tasks, Chores, or Assignments**
- **DE 3.3: Difficult Tasks, Chores, or Assignments**
- **DE 3.4: Aversive Physical Stimuli or Event**

GENERAL DESCRIPTION

Direct escape (DE) functions involve behavior that effectively and efficiently terminates or avoids an aversive (undesired) activity or event (in a direct, nonsocially mediated manner). Such an activity is sufficiently aversive at that particular point in time for escape from such to have value (compared to other possible MCs); hence, an MC exists for such activities/events. All three examples in Table 1.12, despite having different behavioral topographies, have the same function (i.e., getting away from an unpleasant social situation), under a given MC.

Table 1.12: Examples of DE functions

MC	Behavior	Function of behavior
Time to begin strenuous exercising in PE class, following preferred activity	Hides in bathroom	Avoids exercises for some period of time
Asked to begin strenuous exercising in PE class	Runs out of gymnasium	Avoids exercises for some period of time
Asked to begin jumping jacks in PE class	After doing a few jumping jacks, stops and sits down	Directly terminates involvement for some period of time

DE behaviors do not produce their effects via someone else terminating (or postponing) the aversive events or situations. Their escape or avoidance of these situations results directly from the behavior itself. Hence, behaviors that entail leaving the area are often the behavioral mechanism for such escape functions. Contrast this function with socially mediated escape (SME) functions where the form of behavior is irrelevant; the social environment determines what behavior results in the removal of the aversive condition or situation.

DE 3.1: UNPLEASANT SOCIAL SITUATIONS

Under Motivating Conditions (MC), problem target behavior(s) is effective in terminating or postponing/avoiding unpleasant social situations. The following areas can constitute such social situations: simple compliance with adult requests, criticism (with respect to behavior, work performance, or criticism of appearance by peers), adult disapproval statements, social interactions (e.g., interactions with a certain peer or adult, having an argument, having a large number of people in a room, having just a few people in a room, lengthy conversations), and threatened or implemented intended punishment consequences for behavior (removal to time-out, removal of privileges, fines involving points, etc.).

MC for DE 3.1

The presence (or impending presentation) of an unpleasant social situation for the individual *at that point in time* creates a *sufficient* state of aversion that (a) termination/removal of the situation becomes more valued (compared to other present or impending aversive events or access to desired items/activities) and (b) behaviors that are effective in terminating (or avoiding) such become more probable at that point in time.

Diagnostic Criteria

1. Presence of MC for DE 3.1.
2. Target problem behavior(s) is more effective/efficient than other behaviors at directly terminating such undesired situations under the MC (i.e., there exists a far greater reliable relation between target behavior and terminating such aversive activities than other behaviors; Table 1.13).

Table 1.13: Example 1 of unpleasant social situation

MC	Behavior	Result on desired outcome	Future likelihood of behavior (under MC)
1:20 p.m. Criticized for drawing a house that did not have a roof	1:20 p.m. "I will not draw anymore if you do not like my art work!"	Teacher continues criticism (i.e., "You need to put a roof on the house, to make it a good drawing.")	
	1:21 p.m. Leaves class crying	Directly terminates further criticism	More likely in the future if such behavior is left unfettered

Explanation: Note that leaving the area directly terminates any further teacher reflection on the student's work (escape function). But such behavior also sets up an aversive condition for the teacher. The teacher will be less likely to criticize this student's work in the future because of its potential result on student behavior (leaving the class crying). Hence, such behavior can also involve an avoidance function, by making teacher criticism less probable (Table 1.14).

Table 1.14: Example 2 of unpleasant social situation

MC	Behavior	Result on desired outcome	Future likelihood of behavior (Under MC)
3:00 p.m. Being taken to time out (TO) for hitting another child on playground	3:00 p.m. "I did not do it!"	Not effective; adult recess supervisor continues to march student to time out	
	3:00 p.m. Falls to ground	After waiting a few minutes, adult leaves area and child goes back to playground	More likely the next time, time-out being effected

Explanation: Complaining immediately had little effect on the progression to time-out. However, falling to the ground does work, and immediately terminates the progression to time-out. It further resulted in the avoidance of being in the time out area, as the recess supervisor left the child after a few minutes. Consider this: The more a child weighs, the more effective such a behavior is. The ability of an adult to lift someone off the ground diminishes with an increased weight of the target child. This illustrates how some behaviors are effective in escaping and/or avoiding mild to moderate consequences.

Trigger Analysis Procedures

■ If the unpleasant social situation involves peers, simply conduct a naturalistic observation of the phenomenon, since involving others in a trigger analysis simulation could provoke considerable logistical and privacy issues. If you are dealing with social situations involving a teacher or adult (e.g., criticism of work assignment), then proceed with the following steps for the trigger analysis.

■ Always obtain written consent to perform these tests as part of the assessment process for problem behaviors.

■ Set a ceiling limit for the duration of the trial (e.g., 5 minutes, 10 minutes; if the initial time ceiling is insufficient, increase it in subsequent trials and use that data only; delete prior data from previous ceiling).

■ If a dangerous behavior (leaving the area while under the supervision of school staff may constitute a significant problem) is the target problem, then select a precursor behavior, upon which the unpleasant social situation will be immediately removed contingently.

■ To induce the aversive condition, present a form of the social situation (e.g., criticize some aspect of the student's work or behavior, ask the student to comply with a simple request).

■ When the target behavior occurs, the trial ends at that point.

■ Record a plus if the target behavior (or precursor behavior) occurs within the time limit (i.e., before the ceiling) or a minus if it did not.

■ Provide a minimum (over several days) of five trials or until a pattern emerges, that is, most occurrences or nonoccurrences.

Divergent Validity: *See* Adult/Staff Attention: Trigger Analysis

Conduct the attention trigger analysis as a control (contrast) condition for the aforementioned assessment of DE 3.1 category diagnostic function.

If the data collected in this divergent validity test show a low or zero level of target behavior (or precursor if that was selected for analysis aforementioned), divergent validity is established. One can put greater confidence in the selection of the DE 3.1 function. If the rate of the target behavior is high under this divergent validity test, then a DE 3.1 seems unlikely. Rather, an SMA 2.1: Adult/Staff Attention should be entertained. Further anecdotal evidence during the divergent validity test for an SMA 2.1 classification being operative would be the following observation: The target behavior stops immediately or shortly after adult attention is given.

Under MCs, problem target behavior(s) is effective in directly terminating or postponing/avoiding lengthy tasks, chores, or assignments.

MC for DE 3.2

The presence (or impending presentation) of a task, chore, or instructional assignment for the individual *at that point in time* creates a *sufficient* state of aversion that (a) termination/removal of the ongoing tasks, chores, or instructional assignment becomes more valued (compared to other present or impending aversive events or access to desired items/activities) and (b) behaviors that are effective in terminating (or avoiding) such aversive lengthy tasks, assignments become more probable at that point in time.

DE behaviors do not produce their effects via someone else terminating (or postponing) the task or chore. Escape or avoidance of tasks, chores, and/or assignments is a direct result of the behavior. Hence, behaviors that entail leaving the area are often the mechanism for such escape functions. Contrast this function with SME functions where the form of behavior is irrelevant; the social environment determines what behavior results in the removal of the task or chore.

Diagnostic Criteria

1. Presence of MC for DE 3.2.
2. Lengthy tasks, chores, and/or assignments are often embodied in the practice of presenting more work to students contingent upon finishing their initial assigned work (see the "Case of the Wacky Contingencies" in Chapter 3 of Cipani & Schock, 2011). This is often the case where an instructional session lasts for a fixed period of time; hence, completing work results in more of the same, not a transfer to a more preferred activity. Providing more nonpreferred work only increases the MC at that point in time.
3. Target problem behavior(s) is more effective/efficient than other behaviors at terminating lengthy aversive tasks, chores, or instructional assignments under the MC (i.e., there is a far greater reliable relation between target behavior and terminating such aversive activities, as opposed to other behaviors; Tables 1.15 and 1.16).

Table 1.15: Example 1 of lengthy task, chore, or instruction

MC	Behavior	Result on desired outcome	Future likelihood of behavior (under MC)
8:45 a.m. Math period begins; given a seat assignment to complete 25 problems involving fractions	8:45 a.m. Student works for about 12 minutes, finishes all 25 problems	Not effective at terminating math seat work, given more problems to do since there is still plenty of time left	
	8:57 a.m. Begins working on the new assignment; halfway through complains about the amount of work	Complaining results only in being told to go back to desk and finish paper	
	9:12 a.m. After continuing to work, runs out of classroom	Effective, terminates engagement with math assignment at that point	Such unauthorized leaving of area (often called "running") more likely

Explanation: It is important to note that, unfortunately, completing the first assignment results in getting more! Hence, task engagement does not produce a more preferred activity. Instead, it results in more of the same.[11] Therefore, another behavior may be required for such a stimulus change. Regrettably, running out of the classroom

---

11   Think of what life in many classrooms would be like if one's performance on assignments mattered (in terms of accessing more preferred events instead of more of the same)! Instead, finishing one's initial assignment translates to getting more work to do, which I (Ennio Cipani) refer to as the "Wacky Contingency" (Cipani & Schock, 2011).

immediately results in disengagement with materials for some period of time.

When such a behavior becomes frequent, as a result of its ability to terminate task engagement, a referral for a serious management problem will be made. If the plan developed entails curtailing such attempts to leave the classroom, it is possible that other behaviors that produce such a desired outcome develop and become more probable (see SMA and SME Functions).

Table 1.16: Example 2 of lengthy task, chore, or instruction

MC	Behavior	Result on desired outcome	Future likelihood of behavior (under MC)
2:05 p.m. Student is in the library listening to the librarian talk about the Dewey Decimal system	2:05 p.m. Listens for 20 minutes without incident	None	
	2:25 p.m. With presentation still ongoing, student gets up to engage in some other activity	Not allowed, told to sit down and wait for the librarian to finish presentation	
	2:27 p.m.	Looks down at foot and begins untying shoe laces	Immediate break from listening; more likely in future

Explanation: The librarian's presentation, which posed no problem for a while, does become aversive to this student about 20 minutes into the lecture. If the presentation had stopped at 2:20 p.m., the student would not have proceeded to engage in either the complaining or the disruptive behavior. Engaging in an activity with one's shoes does the trick: immediate break. Consider that such passive off-task behaviors are an immediate termination in the task or listening activity, hence their function is direct. It is also the manner in which all of us disengage from a task (e.g., reading, studying) when the length of continuous engaged time becomes onerous and we desire a break from such. It becomes a management problem when the frequency/duration of off-task behaviors becomes excessive in the classroom. Special note for this diagnostic category test:

Unique to this function, category of DE 3.2 is the stipulation that the aversive condition of task presentation is the length of the instructional session (e.g., seatwork, lecture; implying that the individual can perform the task accurately and fluently). Hence, a diagnosis of DE 3.3: escape from difficult instruction should be ruled out first. *Therefore, one should first conduct the trigger analysis test for DE 3.3: escape from instruction: difficult task, assignment, or chores.* If the target behavior appears, select that classification as the probable function (and in fact such an instructional mismatch should be addressed first). If the target behavior does not appear within the ceiling (or the precursor) for a DE 3.3 test, then proceed to test the DE 3.2 diagnostic category.

Trigger Analysis Procedures

- Set a ceiling limit for the duration of the trial (e.g., 35 minutes; if the initial time ceiling is insufficient, increase it in subsequent trials and use that data only; delete prior data from previous ceiling). Since one is testing the time duration aspect of the task, the ceiling should be longer than the other trigger analyses to encompass the point at which the MC is achieved.
- Always obtain written consent to perform these tests as part of the assessment process for problem behaviors.
- If a dangerous behavior (leaving the area while under the supervision of school staff may constitute a significant problem) is the target problem, then select a precursor behavior, upon which task will be immediately removed contingently.
- To induce the aversive condition, continue presenting lengthy tasks until the ceiling limit is reached.
- When the target behavior occurs, the trial ends at that point.
- Record a plus if the target behavior (or precursor behavior) occurs within the time limit (i.e., before the ceiling) or a minus if it did not.
- Provide a minimum (over several days) of five trials or until a pattern emerges, that is, most occurrences or nonoccurrences.

Divergent Validity: Short Defined Task Assignment

Unique to this function, category of DE 3.2 is the stipulation that the aversive condition of task presentation is the length of the instructional session (e.g., seatwork, lecture; and not difficulty of material/content). Perform the following trigger analysis for short defined tasks (delineated as follows).

- Set a ceiling limit for the short duration of the trial (e.g., 3 minutes).
- Always obtain written consent to perform these tests as part of the assessment process for problem behaviors.
- Present a defined, but short task, chore, or instructional content/material representative of the grade level of the student's current curriculum (remember, you should have first ruled out difficulty of the material as the MC). Prompt the student to initiate work by saying, "Here are just a few problems for you to work on. When you have finished this task, you can take a 5- to 10-minute break from work (at one's seat)."
- If the student finishes the task before the ceiling limit, end the trial and record a minus for that trial.
- If the target or precursor behavior occurs, the task will be immediately removed and the test trial ends.
- Record a plus if the target behavior (or precursor behavior) occurs within the time limit (i.e., before the ceiling) or a minus if it did not.
- Provide a minimum (over several days) of five trials or until a pattern emerges (i.e., most occurrences or nonoccurrences).

If the data collected in this divergent validity test show a low or zero level of target behavior (or precursor if that was selected for analysis aforementioned), divergent validity is established. One can put greater confidence in the selection of the DE 3.2 function. If the rate of the target behavior is high under this divergent validity test, then another function would seem more plausible.

Under MCs, problem target behavior(s) is effective in terminating, postponing, or avoiding difficult tasks, chores, or assignments.

MC for DE 3.3

The presence (or impending presentation) of a difficult task, chore, or instructional assignment for the individual *at that point in time* creates a *sufficient* state of aversion that (a) termination/removal of the ongoing difficult tasks, chores, or instructional assignments become more valued (compared to other present or impending aversive events or access to desired items/activities) and (b) behaviors that are directly effective in terminating (or avoiding) such become more probable at that point in time.

Diagnostic Criteria
1. Presence of MC for DE 3.3.
2. Tasks and/or instructional assignments that constitute a difficult condition (and hence aversive) for the individual can be determined initially by examining the person's standardized test scores in the content area versus the actual grade level material at which the person is required to perform. For example, someone's reading grade level on an achievement test is at beginning second grade. However, this student is placed in a fifth-grade mainstream class. This creates an "instructional mismatch" or performance discrepancy. The greater the performance discrepancy (e.g., one grade level versus four grade levels), the greater the state of aversion produced.
3. Target problem behavior(s) is more effective/efficient than other behaviors at terminating difficult aversive tasks, chores, or instructional assignments (i.e., there is a far greater reliable relation between target behavior and terminating such aversive activities, as opposed to other behaviors). If DE behavior is unencumbered, such will occur under the MC relative to other behaviors that do not directly produce escape (Tables 1.17 and 1.18).

Table 1.17: Example 1 of difficult task, chore, or instruction

MC	Behavior	Result on desired outcome	Future likelihood of behavior (under MC)
10:10 a.m. Presented with difficult math assignment	10:10 a.m. "I cannot do this."	None	
	10:12 a.m. Walks out of classroom	Effective immediately; postponement of work depends on how quickly student is returned to classroom[12]	If there is no effort to bring student back (for whatever reason), such behavior is likely in future under difficult math work

Explanation: Under the MC of being presented with difficult math seatwork, the student's verbal request to have the assignment changed is ineffective. Hence, such comments are less likely in the future. However, leaving the classroom does produce the desired effect: termination of work assignment. Hopefully, if such behavior persists over time, particularly with respect to this curriculum area, the task difficulty issue will be addressed. Altering that aversive event would address the student leaving the class under this MC for the long term. The student's capability to be competent in the presented instructional curriculum would take care of this problem.

---

12   Of course, the solution to this type of function is to address the instructional mismatch.

Table 1.18: Example 2 of difficult task, chore, or instruction

MC	Behavior	Result on desired outcome	Future likelihood of behavior (under MC)
11:08 a.m. Asked to read aloud a passage from a fourth-grade text (let's assume current achievement level is that of second grade)	11:08 a.m. Walks out of class	Effective	If "ignored," such behavior will become more prevalent—but staff should address instructional mismatch!

Explanation: Under the MC of being presented an oral reading task that is two grade levels above the student's current capability, leaving the classroom does produce the desired outcome. This performance discrepancy should seem to be an obvious explanation for this student's behavior[13]. Hopefully, the instructional mismatch will be addressed sooner rather than later.

Trigger Analysis Procedures

- Set a ceiling limit for the duration of the trial (e.g., 5 minutes, 10 minutes). Since one is testing the difficulty aspect of the task/assignment, the ceiling need not be that long to encompass the point at which the MC is achieved.
- Always obtain written consent to perform these tests as part of the assessment process for problem behaviors.
- If a dangerous behavior (leaving the area while under the supervision of school staff may constitute a significant problem) is the target problem, then select a precursor behavior, upon which task will be immediately removed contingently.
- Present the difficult task, chore, or instructional content/material. Prompt the student to initiate work.
- When the target (or precursor) behavior occurs, the trial ends at that point. The difficult task will be immediately removed contingently and replaced with a much easier task (e.g., some

---

13   Too often, this instructional mismatch is the MC for many student's problem behavior.

material that is one to two grade levels below the student's achievement level).

- Record a plus if the target behavior (or precursor behavior) occurs within the time limit (i.e., before the ceiling) or a minus if it did not.
- Provide a minimum (over several days) of five trials or until a pattern emerges (i.e., most occurrences or nonoccurrences).

Divergent Validity: Easy Tasks

Unique to this function, category of DE 3.3 is the stipulation that the aversive condition of task presentation is the difficulty of the instructional session, for example, seatwork, lecture. Therefore, there is an implication that the individual can accurately and fluently perform easier tasks. To test the veracity of this contention, conduct the following trigger analysis procedures for easy tasks (delineated as follows).

- Set a ceiling limit for the duration of the trial (e.g., 5 minutes, 10 minutes).
- Always obtain written consent to perform these tests as part of the assessment process for problem behaviors.
- Present the easy task, chore, or instructional content/material. The material presented should be one to two grade levels below the student's achievement level in the designated content area. Prompt the student to initiate work.
- With the target or precursor behavior occurring, the easy task will be immediately removed contingently and replaced with a neutral activity (e.g., doing nothing until ceiling duration limit is reached).
- Record a plus if the target behavior (or precursor behavior) occurs within the time limit (i.e., before the ceiling) or a minus if it did not.
- Provide a minimum (over several days) of five trials or until a pattern emerges, that is, most occurrences or nonoccurrences.

If the data collected in this divergent validity test show a low or zero level of target behavior (or precursor if that was selected for analysis aforementioned), divergent validity is established. If divergent validity is not obtained, conduct further investigations into the problem behavior's function.

Under MCs, problem target behavior(s) is effective in directly terminating, or avoiding aversive physical stimuli. Such aversive physical stimuli can include any items or events (nonsocial aspect of an event) that produce avoidance behavior (engender a "fear" reaction when confronted with such). Sensations such as visual, auditory, gustatory, and so on, can also be stimuli that generate escape or avoidance behavior.

MC for DE 3.4

The presence (or impending presentation) of aversive stimuli for the individual *at that point in time* creates a *sufficient* state of aversion that: (a) the termination/removal of the aversive stimuli become more valued (compared to other present or impending aversive events or access to desired items/activities) and (b) behaviors that are effective in terminating (or avoiding) such become more probable at that point in time.

Diagnostic Criteria
1. Presence of MC for DE 3.4.
2. Target problem behavior(s) is more effective/efficient than other behaviors at terminating aversive physical stimuli (i.e., there is a far greater reliable relation between target behavior and terminating such aversive activities, as opposed to other behaviors).

Aversive Physical Stimuli/Event: Obviously, what is aversive to one individual may not be to someone else. Hence, the selection of the aversive stimulus should be made by examining anecdotally the individual's response to certain stimuli. What is a warm room to some is a cool room (temperature wise) to others. When a physical stimulus generates avoidance behavior, select this as an MC for this category (Tables 1.19 and 1.20).

Table 1.19: Example 1 of aversive stimuli

MC	Behavior	Result on desired outcome	Future likelihood of behavior (under MC)
2:09 p.m. Too hot in the room	2:09 p.m. Goes to thermostat and turns down the temperature to 6°	Effective	What many people have learned to do!

Explanation: Altering the temperature in the room is a pretty obvious solution. Another possible behavior might be to leave from a room to another room, that is, one with air conditioning.

Table 1.20: Example 2 of aversive stimuli

MC	Behavior	Result on desired outcome	Future likelihood of behavior (under MC)
7:59 a.m. Staff put a shirt on student that does not fit well (but not discernible to them)	8:09 a.m. Cries for several minutes and tries to take shirt off	Not effective	
	8:16 a.m. Runs to bathroom and tears off shirt	No more unfitted shirt! Immediate loss of uncomfortable attire. Must be given another one.	Hopefully, some other behavior that communicates to staff the student's need will be developed

Explanation: For some students who do not have the verbal skills to communicate to others such an aversive condition, such extreme behaviors are the only manner of terminating such a condition. Note that crying and mild attempts to take the shirt off were met by staff interventions only to keep the shirt on the student. Hence, leaving the area so that he could remove the shirt unencumbered becomes the only viable alternative.

Trigger Analysis Procedures

- Conduct this test only if the designated aversive stimuli do not present significant danger or threat to the individual. If such is the case, one should collect anecdotal and/or direct observation data when phenomenon occurs naturally. If the aversive physical stimuli do not constitute such a danger or threat, follow the steps below.
- Always obtain written consent to perform these tests as part of the assessment process for problem behaviors.
- Set a ceiling limit for the duration of the trial, for example, 5 minutes, 10 minutes, (if the initial time ceiling is insufficient, increase it in subsequent trials and use that data only; delete prior data from previous ceiling).
- If a dangerous behavior (to self, property, or others) is the target problem, then select a precursor behavior, upon which the aversive stimulus will be immediately removed contingently.
- Present the aversive physical stimulus.
- Record a plus if the target behavior (or precursor behavior) occurs within the time limit (i.e., before the ceiling) or a minus if it did not.
- Provide a minimum (over several days) of five trials or until a pattern emerges, that is, most occurrences or nonoccurrences.

Divergent Validity: *See* Adult Attention: Trigger Analysis Procedures

Conduct the attention trigger analysis as a control (contrast) condition for the above test of escape from aversive physical stimuli function.

If the data collected in this divergent validity test show a low or zero level of target behavior (or precursor if that was selected for analysis aforementioned), divergent validity is established. One can put greater confidence in the selection of the DE 4.4 function. If the rate of the target behavior is high under this divergent validity test, then a DE 4.4 category seems unlikely. Rather, an SMA 2.1: Adult/Staff Attention should be entertained. Further anecdotal evidence during the divergent validity test for an SMA 2.1 classification being operative would be the following observation: The target behavior stops immediately or shortly after adult attention is given.

SOCIALLY MEDIATED ESCAPE (SME 4.0) FUNCTIONS

- SME 4.1: Unpleasant Social Situations
- SME 4.2: Lengthy Tasks, Chores, or Assignments
- SME 4.3: Difficult Tasks, Chores, or Assignments
- SME 4.4: Aversive Physical Stimuli or Event

GENERAL DESCRIPTION

Socially mediated escape functions involve behavior that effectively and efficiently terminates or avoids an aversive (undesired) activity or event (through someone's acting on such behavior). Such an activity is sufficiently aversive at that particular point in time for escape from such to have value (relative to other possible MCs); hence, an MC becomes operable for such activities/events. All three following examples, despite having different behavioral topographies, have the same function (i.e., getting away from an unpleasant social situation), under a given MC (Table 1.21).

Table 1.21: Examples of SME functions

MC	Behavior	Function of behavior
Asked to begin strenuous exercising in PE class	Complains	Teacher provides an alternate activity, student gets out of doing strenuous exercises
Asked to begin strenuous exercising in PE class	After doing two jumping jacks, student makes rude comment, "Take your jumping jacks and $##%%!"	Gets sent to the principal's office for the remainder of the period
Asked to begin jumping jacks in PE class	Hits self a number of times in the face	Teacher stops student from hitting self, moves student away from activity (terminates exercise)

Under motivating conditions (MC), problem target behavior(s) is effective in terminating or postponing/avoiding unpleasant social situations by the action of someone else (i.e., social mediation). The following areas can constitute such social situations: simple compliance with adult requests, criticism (with respect to behavior, work performance, or criticism of appearance by peers), adult disapproval statements, social interactions (e.g., interactions with a certain peer or adult, having an argument, having a large number of people in a room, having just a few people in a room, lengthy conversations), and threatened or implemented intended punishment consequences for behavior (removal to time-out, removal of privileges, fines involving points, etc.).

MC for SME 4.1
The presence (or impending presentation) of an unpleasant social situation for the individual *at that point in time* creates a *sufficient* state of aversion that (a) termination/removal of the situation becomes more valued (compared to other present or impending aversive events or access to desired items/activities) and (b) behaviors that are effective in terminating (or avoiding) such become more probable at that point in time.

Diagnostic Criteria
1. Presence of MC for SME 4.1.
2. Target problem behavior(s) is more effective/efficient than other behaviors at terminating such undesired situations under the MC, that is, there exists a far greater reliable relation between target behavior and terminating such aversive activities than other behaviors.
3. Presence of person(s) who has a history of terminating such situations under the specific MC for target problem behaviors (person is discriminative for removal or postponement of such aversive situations for such behaviors; Tables 1.22 and 1.23).

Table 1.22: Example 1 of unpleasant social situation

MC	Behavior	Result on desired outcome	Future likelihood of behavior (under MC)
Criticized for drawing a house that did not have a roof	"I will not draw anymore if you do not like my art work!"	Person apologizes	Very likely if such produces apology and avoids future criticism

Explanation: Note that the uncouth comment by the student results in an apology. Hence, the ceasing of criticism is an initial effect of such a form of behavior. But there is an additional benefit of such a functional behavior. It also serves to make criticism less likely in the future; the teacher avoids giving criticism as a result of its relation to the dramatic verbal behavior that can follow.

Table 1.23: Example 2 of unpleasant social situation

MC	Behavior	Result on desired outcome	Future likelihood of behavior (under MC)
3:00 p.m. Being taken to TO for hitting another child on playground	3:00 p.m. "I did not do it!"	Not effective; adult recess supervisor continues to guide student to TO	
	3:00 p.m. Spits at supervisor	Terminates TO. The supervisor is stunned, releases student, and reports the incident to principal	More likely the next time when TO is attempted (especially if spitting incident is not dealt with effectively)

Explanation: Complaining immediately had little effect on the transport to time-out. However, note that the next behavior (spitting) is effective in terminating the time-out. Spitting on staff will halt the progression to time-out for a while. Once again, such an extreme reaction over time will become a functional mechanism to reduce the frequency of time-outs (when needed). After all, who wants to get spit on, when one can avoid such! "Why bother," becomes the suitable mantra.

Trigger Analysis Procedures

- If the unpleasant social situation involves peers, simply conduct a naturalistic observation of the phenomenon, since involving others in a trigger analysis simulation could provoke considerable logistical and privacy issues. If you are dealing with social situations involving a teacher or adult (e.g., criticism of work assignment), then proceed with the following steps for the trigger analysis.
- Always obtain written consent to perform these tests as part of the assessment process for problem behaviors.
- Set a ceiling limit for the duration of the trial (e.g., 5 minutes, 10 minutes; if the initial time ceiling is insufficient, increase it in subsequent trials and use that data only; delete prior data from previous ceiling).
- If a dangerous behavior (to self, property, or others) is the target problem, then select a precursor behavior, upon which the unpleasant social situation will be immediately removed contingently.
- To induce the aversive condition, present a form of the social situation, for example, criticize some aspect of the student's work or behavior.
- When the target behavior occurs, cease the situation (e.g., stop criticizing the student and walk away).
- Record a plus if the target behavior (or precursor behavior) occurs within the time limit (i.e., before the ceiling) or a minus if it did not.
- Provide a minimum (over several days) of five trials or until a pattern emerges (i.e., most occurrences or nonoccurrences).

Divergent Validity: *See* Adult Attention: Trigger Analysis

Conduct the attention trigger analysis as a control (contrast) condition for the above test of escape from unpleasant social situation category.

If the data collected in this divergent validity test show a low or zero level of target behavior (or precursor if that was selected for analysis aforementioned), divergent validity is established. One can put greater confidence in the selection of the SME 4.1 function. If the rate of the target behavior is high under this divergent validity test, then an SME 4.1 seems unlikely. Rather, an SMA 2.1: Adult/Staff Attention should be entertained. Further anecdotal evidence during the divergent validity test for an SMA 2.1 classification being operative would be the following observation: The target behavior stops immediately or shortly after adult attention is given.

SME 4.2: LENGTHY TASKS, CHORES, OR ASSIGNMENTS

Under MCs, problem target behavior(s) is effective in terminating or postponing/avoiding lengthy tasks, chores, or instructional assignments by the action of someone else, that is, social mediation.

MC for SME 4.2

The presence (or impending presentation) of a task, chore, or instructional assignment for the individual *at that point in time* creates a *sufficient* state of aversion that (a) termination/removal of the ongoing tasks, chores, or instructional assignments becomes more valued (compared to other present or impending aversive events or access to desired items/activities) and (b) behaviors that are effective in terminating (or avoiding) such become more probable at that point in time.

Diagnostic Criteria

1. Presence of MC for SME 4.2.
2. Lengthy tasks and/or assignments are often mirrored in the practice of presenting more work to students contingent upon finishing their initial assigned work (see the "Case of the Wacky Contingencies" in Chapter 3 of Cipani & Schock, 2011). This is often the circumstance where an instructional session lasts for a fixed period of time; hence, completing work results in more of the same, not a transfer to a more preferred activity. Providing more nonpreferred work only increases the MC at that point in time.
3. Target problem behavior(s) is more effective/efficient than other behaviors at terminating lengthy aversive tasks, chores, or assignments (i.e., there is a far greater reliable relation between target behavior and terminating such aversive activities, as opposed to other behaviors).
4. Presence of person(s) who has a history of terminating lengthy tasks/chores or instructional assignments under the specific MC for target problem behaviors (person is discriminative for task removal or postponement for such behaviors; Tables 1.24 and 1.25).

Table 1.24: Example 1 of lengthy task, chore, or instruction

MC	Behavior	Result on desired outcome	Future likelihood of behavior (under MC)
8:45 a.m. Math period begins; given a seat assignment to complete 25 problems involving fractions	8:45 a.m. Student works for about 12 minutes, finishes all 25 problems	Given an additional assignment	
	9:18 a.m. About halfway through this assignment, complains about the amount of work	Complaining only results in being told to go back to the desk and finish	
	9:22 a.m. Throws pencil on floor—told to go sit in principal's office	Effective, ends math assignment at that point	Such disruptive behavior more likely, especially since doing some amount of work is ineffectual

Explanation: When completing the assigned work results in getting more, engaging in disruptive behavior succeeds in getting the student kicked out of class (sans math assignment)! It is important to note that this student worked for some period of time (almost half an hour). Yet a change to a more preferred instructional task (or other activity) was not effected! One should conclude that disruptive behaviors seem to be the manner in which relatively lengthy assignments are ceased in this hypothetical class.

Table 1.25: Example 2 of lengthy task, chore, or instruction

MC	Behavior	Result on desired outcome	Future likelihood of behavior (under MC)
2:05 p.m. Student is in library, listening to the librarian talk about the Dewey Decimal system	2:05 p.m. Listens for 20 minutes without incident	None	
	2:25 p.m. With presentation still ongoing, student asks if he can leave area, "I am bored."	Not allowed; told to continue listening to this important information	
	2:27 p.m. Hits classmate sitting next to him	Told to leave group and go outside and wait	Disruptive behaviors become more likely in future

Explanation: The librarian's presentation, which posed no problem for a while, does become aversive to this student about 20 minutes into the lecture. If the presentation had stopped at 2:20 p.m., the student would not have proceeded to engage in either the complaining or the disruptive behavior. While requesting to leave does not result in getting to leave, hitting a classmate does work! Enough said.

Special note for this diagnostic category test:

Unique to this function, category of SME 4.2 is the stipulation that the aversive condition of task presentation is the length of the instructional session, for example, seatwork, lecture (implying that the individual can perform the task accurately and fluently). Hence, a diagnosis of SME 4.3: escape from difficult instruction should be ruled out first. *Therefore, one should first conduct the test for escape from instruction: difficult task, assignment, or chores.* If the target behavior appears, select that classification as the probable function (and in fact such an instructional mismatch should be addressed first). If the target behavior does not appear within the ceiling (or the precursor) for a SME 4.3 test, then proceed to test the SME 4.2 diagnostic category (instructions given earlier).

Trigger Analysis Procedures

- Set a ceiling limit for the duration of the trial, for example, 35 minutes (if the initial time ceiling is insufficient, increase it in subsequent trials and use that data only; delete prior data from previous ceiling). Since one is testing the lengthy aspect of the task, the ceiling should be longer than the other trigger analyses to encompass the point at which the MC is achieved.
- Always obtain written consent to perform these tests as part of the assessment process for problem behaviors.
- If a dangerous behavior (to self, property, or others) is the target problem, then select a precursor behavior, upon which task will be immediately removed contingently.
- To induce the aversive condition, continue presenting the tasks until the ceiling limit is reached.
- When the target behavior occurs, end the trial. Immediately remove the task and have the individual wait a few minutes before entering another (more preferred activity); the trial ends at that point.
- Record a plus if the target behavior (or precursor behavior) occurs within the time limit (i.e., before the ceiling) or a minus if it did not.
- Provide a minimum (over several days) of five trials or until a pattern emerges, for example, most occurrences or nonoccurrences.

Divergent Validity: Short Defined Task Assignment

Unique to this function, category of SME 4.2 is the stipulation that the aversive condition of task presentation is the length of the instructional session (e.g., seatwork, lecture; and not difficulty of material/content). Perform the following trigger analysis for short defined tasks (delineated as follows).

- Set a ceiling limit for the short duration of the trial (e.g., 3 minutes).
- Always obtain written consent to perform these tests as part of the assessment process for problem behaviors.

- Present a defined, but short task, chore, or instructional content/ material representative of the grade level of the student's current curriculum (remember, you should have first ruled out difficulty of the material as the MC). Prompt the student to initiate work by saying, "Here are just a few problems for you to work on. When you have finished this task, you can take a 5- to 10-minute break from work (at one's seat)."
- If the student finishes the task before the ceiling limit, end the trial and record a minus for that trial.
- If the target or precursor behavior occurs, the task will be immediately removed and the test trial ends.
- Record a plus if the target behavior (or precursor behavior) occurs within the time limit (i.e., before the ceiling) or a minus if it did not.
- Provide a minimum (over several days) of five trials or until a pattern emerges (i.e., most occurrences or nonoccurrences).

If the data collected in this divergent validity test show a low or zero level of target behavior (or precursor if that was selected for analysis aforementioned), divergent validity is established. One can put greater confidence in the selection of the SME 4.2 function. If the rate of the target behavior is high under this divergent validity test, then another function would seem more plausible.

Under MCs, problem target behavior(s) is effective in terminating or postponing or avoiding difficult tasks, chores, or assignments by the action of someone else, that is, social mediation.

MC for SME 4.3

The presence (or impending presentation) of a difficult task, chore, or instructional assignment for the individual *at that point in time* creates a *sufficient* state of aversion that (a) termination/removal of the ongoing difficult tasks, chores, or instructional assignments become more valued (compared to other present or impending aversive events or access to desired items/activities) and (b) behaviors that are effective in terminating (or avoiding) such become more probable at that point in time.

Diagnostic Criteria
1. Presence of MC for SME 4.3.
2. Tasks and/or assignments that constitute a difficult condition (and hence aversive) for the individual can be determined initially by examining the person's standardized test scores in the content area versus the actual grade level material at which the person is required to perform. For example, someone's reading grade level on an achievement test is at beginning second grade. However, this student is placed in a fifth-grade mainstream class. This creates an "instructional mismatch" or performance discrepancy. The greater the performance discrepancy (e.g., one grade level versus four grade levels), the greater the state of aversion produced.
3. Target problem behavior(s) are more effective/efficient than other behaviors at terminating difficult aversive tasks, chores, instructional assignments under the MC (i.e., there is a far greater reliable relation between target behavior and terminating such aversive activities, as opposed to other behaviors).
4. Presence of person(s) who has a history of terminating difficult tasks, chores, or instructional assignments under the specific MC for target problem behaviors (person is discriminative for task removal or postponement for such behaviors). Such removal can be either in the form of removal of instruction (but then test for SME 4.2) or the provision of easier material or assignments (Tables 1.26 and 1.27).

Table 1.26: Example 1 of difficult task, chore, or instruction

MC	Behavior	Result on desired outcome	Future likelihood of behavior (under MC)
10:10 a.m. Present difficult math seat assignment	10:10 a.m. "I cannot do this."	None	
	10:12 a.m. "This is really hard. How do you expect me to do this?"	None	
	10:17 a.m. Puts a big X across the paper and throws it on the floor	Is given a different, easier assignment after some admonishment	

Explanation: Under the MC of being presented with difficult math seatwork, two verbal requests to have the assignment changed are ineffective. Hence, such comments are less likely in the future. However, marking up the paper and throwing it on the floor does produce an easier task assignment. As is evident from these scenarios, the student is more likely to engage in a more demonstrative protest when faced with such difficult work in the future, as such behaviors are more likely to result in a removal of the difficult assignment and introduction of easier work.

Table 1.27: Example 2 of difficult task, chore, or instruction

MC	Behavior	Result on desired outcome	Future likelihood of behavior (under MC)
11:08 a.m. Asked to read aloud a passage from a fourth-grade text (let's assume current achievement level is first grade)	11:08 a.m. Hides under desk in his seat	"Okay Bobby, I am going to go to someone else if you do not sit up in your seat!"	
	11:09 a.m. Still under desk and says "Leave me alone!"	"Okay, Let's have Sarah read those two paragraphs. Bobby, you are not showing appropriate behavior."	

Explanation: Bobby's method of escaping oral reading works! Hide under the seat does not work initially. But adding, "Leave me alone!" does the trick. This scenario represents the MC for the escape behavior as the difficulty of the material. If it was just a matter of finding oral reading an unpleasant event (no problem with reading difficulty), then it would be a SME 4.1: Unpleasant Social Situation function.

Trigger Analysis Procedures

- Set a ceiling limit for the duration of the trial (e.g., 5 minutes, 10 minutes). Since one is testing the difficulty aspect of the task/assignment, the ceiling need not be that long to encompass the point at which the MC is achieved.
- Always obtain written consent to perform these tests as part of the assessment process for problem behaviors.
- If a dangerous behavior (to self, property, or others) is the target problem, then select a precursor behavior, upon which task will be immediately removed contingently.

- Present the difficult task, chore, or instructional content/material. Prompt the student to initiate work.
- When the target (or precursor) behavior occurs, the trial ends at that point. The difficult task will be immediately removed contingently and replaced with a much easier task (e.g., some material that is one to two grade levels below the student's achievement level).
- Record a plus if the target behavior (or precursor behavior) occurs within the time limit (i.e., before the ceiling) or a minus if it did not.
- Provide a minimum (over several days) of five trials or until a pattern emerges, that is, most occurrences or nonoccurrences.

Divergent Validity: Easy Tasks

Unique to this function, category of SME 4.3 is the stipulation that the aversive condition of task presentation is the difficulty of the instructional session (e.g., seatwork, lecture). Therefore, there is an implication that the individual can accurately and fluently perform easier tasks. To test the veracity of this contention, conduct the following trigger analysis procedures for easy tasks (delineated as follows).

- Set a ceiling limit for the duration of the trial (e.g., 5 minutes, 10 minutes).
- Always obtain written consent to perform these tests as part of the assessment process for problem behaviors.
- Present the easy task, chore, or instructional content/material. The material presented should be one to two grade levels below the student's achievement level in the designated content area. Prompt the student to initiate work.
- With the target or precursor behavior occurring, the easy task will be immediately removed contingently and replaced with a neutral activity (doing nothing until ceiling duration limit is reached).
- Record a plus if the target behavior (or precursor behavior) occurs within the time limit (i.e., before the ceiling) or a minus if it did not.
- Provide a minimum (over several days) of five trials or until a pattern emerges, that is, most occurrences or nonoccurrences.

If the data collected in this divergent validity test show a low or zero level of target behavior (or precursor if that was selected for analysis aforementioned), divergent validity is established. If divergent validity is not obtained, conduct further investigations into the problem behavior's function.

SME 4.4: AVERSIVE PHYSICAL STIMULI OR EVENT

Under MCs, problem target behavior(s) is effective in terminating or postponing/avoiding aversive physical stimuli by the action of someone else, that is, social mediation. Such aversive physical stimuli can include any items or events (nonsocial aspect of an event) that produce avoidance behavior (engender a "fear" reaction when confronted with such). Sensations such as visual, auditory, or gustatory can also be stimuli that generate escape or avoidance behavior.

MC for SME 4.4

The presence (or impending presentation) of aversive stimuli for the individual *at that point in time* creates a *sufficient* state of aversion that (a) termination/removal of the aversive stimuli become more valued (compared to other present or impending aversive events or access to desired items/activities) and (b) behaviors that are effective in terminating (or avoiding) such physical stimuli become more probable at that point in time.

Diagnostic Criteria

1. Presence of MC for SME 4.4.
2. Target problem behavior(s) is more effective/efficient than other behaviors at terminating aversive physical stimuli (i.e., there is a far greater reliable relation between target behavior and terminating such aversive activities, as opposed to other behaviors).
3. Presence of person(s) who has a history of terminating the aversive physical stimuli under the specific MC for target problem behaviors (person is discriminative for task removal or postponement for such behaviors).

Aversive Physical Stimuli

Obviously, what is aversive to one individual may not be to someone else. Hence, the selection of the aversive stimulus should be made by examining anecdotally the individual's response to certain stimuli. What is a warm room to some is a cool room (temperature wise) to others. When a stimulus generates avoidance behavior (other than those items, activities, and events that are within the MC parameters of the three previous categories, 4.1, 4.2, and 4.3), select this as an MC for this category (Tables 1.28 and 1.29).

Table 1.28: Example 1 of aversive stimuli

MC	Behavior	Result on desired outcome	Future likelihood of behavior (under MC)
2:09 p.m. Too hot in the room	2:09 p.m. Waves hand in front of face, trying to cool off	Not as effective	
	2:15 p.m. "Can you turn on the air conditioner?"	"Okay, I see it is a little warm here."	Request to alter the thermostat will become more frequent

Explanation: Requesting someone (teacher) to turn on the air conditioner results in the desired effect. This is especially the case when compared to the "try and fan yourself with your hand" method.

Table 1.29: Example 2 of aversive stimuli

MC	Behavior	Result on desired outcome	Future likelihood of behavior (under MC)
2:09 p.m. Told to get into pool	2:09 p.m. Waves hand indicating "No"	Not effective	
	2:15 p.m. Hits staff person who is trying to persuade and mildly escort him into the lower end of pool	Effective, staff person leaves him alone	Hitting someone when they approach you to coax you into the pool will become more likely the next time

Explanation: The student's trepidation and anxiety over the demand to get into the pool reveal the MC: fear of getting into the pool. The student's failure to comply is not a function of the social demand (unpleasant social situation)! It is the desire to not get into or near the pool, whether it is demanded or not. Hence, this classification of SME 4.4 best suits the explanation for hitting the staff person who attempts to guide him into the water.

Trigger Analysis Procedures

- Conduct this test only if the designated aversive stimulus does not present significant danger or threat to the individual. If such is the case, one should collect anecdotal and/or direct observation data when the phenomenon occurs naturally. If the aversive physical stimuli/event do not constitute such a danger or threat, follow the steps as follows.
- Always obtain written consent to perform these tests as part of the assessment process for problem behaviors.
- Set a ceiling limit for the duration of the trial (e.g., 5 minutes, 10 minutes; if the initial time ceiling is insufficient, increase it in subsequent trials and use that data only; delete prior data from previous ceiling).
- If a dangerous behavior (to self, property, or others) is the target problem, then select a precursor behavior, upon which aversive stimulus will be immediately removed contingently.
- When the target behavior occurs, remove the task and have the individual wait a few minutes before entering another (more preferred activity); the trial ends at that point.
- Record a plus if the target behavior (or precursor behavior) occurs within the time limit (i.e., before the ceiling) or a minus if it did not.
- Provide a minimum (over several days) of five trials or until a pattern emerges, that is, most occurrences or nonoccurrences.

Divergent Validity: *See* Adult Attention: Trigger Analysis

Conduct the attention trigger analysis as a control (contrast) condition for the preceding test of escape from aversive physical stimuli function.

If the data collected in this divergent validity test show a low or zero level of target behavior (or precursor if that was selected for analysis aforementioned), divergent validity is established. One can put greater confidence in the selection of the SME 4.4 function. If the rate of the target behavior is high under this divergent validity test, then an SME 4.4 seems unlikely. Rather, an SMA 2.1: Adult/Staff Attention should be entertained. Further anecdotal evidence during the divergent validity test for an SMA 2.1 classification being operative would be the following observation: The target behavior stops immediately or shortly after adult attention is given.

SECTION II: PRACTICE CASE ILLUSTRATIONS

PRACTICE CASE ILLUSTRATIONS

The following hypothetical case presentations provide information regarding the contextual factors surrounding a case with a referral for problem behaviors. The case is presented on the front page, with the answer for self-checking of comprehension on the following back page.

Case 1

Johnny, who has severe intellectual disabilities and is in a wheelchair, hits himself several times a day. He is unable to communicate his needs by vocal speech. Classroom staff claim he is able to use picture icons to communicate (about 15 picture icons on a board). During several observation sessions, you have never seen him use his picture icons for any requesting (or protesting for that matter). But you have observed the following scenario twice during your observation. When he hit himself, the classroom staff told him to, "stop doing that," which was unsuccessful in abating the behavior at that point. Sometime thereafter, while he was still sporadically engaged in hitting himself, someone brought him his juice bottle to drink and his hitting stopped pretty quickly. When he finished drinking the juice, he dropped the bottle on his tray and seemed content.

Question: What is the numeric function, and the function category?

(Answer on next page)

Case 1

The key information leading to this selected function of SMA 2.3: Tangible Reinforcer is the following: (a) reliable relation between behavior and hypothesized reinforcer (juice); (b) behavior seems to be more effective than other behaviors at procuring juice; and (c) the MC seems to be a desire for juice at those times because following the procurement of juice the behavior stops and he drinks the juice provided (by someone, hence socially mediated) at that point.

Note that even though staff gives attention when he hits himself, it has nothing to do with the MC operable at that time. Since he is unable to get juice on his own (possibly due to being in a wheelchair), he must engage in a behavior that obtains juice via staff mediation.

Case 2

In the prior case of Johnny and the self-injury problem behavior, suppose his pointing to the picture of the juice bottle was reliably effective at procuring the juice bottle from staff.

Question: Why would the SMA 2.3 function (Tangible Reinforcer) probably not be operable?

(*Answer on next page*)

Case 2

If you observed Johnny using his communication system to get juice, and such a communicative behavior was effective, then an alternate behavior (and one that is less painful) is available for reinforcement with juice. If such a desirable communication response is effective and efficient (i.e., gets juice fairly readily, without great delay), then that behavior will become highly probable under the MC for tangible reinforcer. Hitting oneself would become less functional; hence less frequent in occurrence when a desire for juice is present.

One note of caution: You should make sure you actually see the student use the communication board to request juice. It is often the case that a claim of a student's proficiency with an alternate communication system is not a currently realized skill. This can be particularly true in that the conditions of training the student to point to the picture of juice are sometimes quite dissimilar from those where the spontaneous need to request is present.

Also, if staff or adults are less efficient or are much less consistent with providing juice when he uses this method in contrast to hitting himself, then such a desirable alternative is not as useful as its undesirable counterpart. Hence, hitting will still occur because of its more straightforward relationship with obtaining juice when desired.

Case 3

Susan, a junior high student in a general education class, yells, "This is stupid!" and the teacher reprimands her in front of the other students. Your involvement has occurred because of this behavior and other similar disrespectful comments to the teacher. The teacher reports these types of comments occur several times a week (data from recall, not actual frequency counts at the time of occurrence).

You have witnessed that when she needs the teacher's help or attention, she calls out and the teacher comes to her.

Question: If SMA 2.1 is not relevant for this scenario, what other socially mediated access function might such derogatory comments recruit? What does the social environment probably do when Susan makes this comment?

(*Answer on next page*)

Case 3

Another very plausible hypothesis about the rude comments function is a diagnostic classification of SMA 2.2: Peer Attention. If teacher attention is not in a state of deprivation due to other behaviors producing such, one must examine the feasibility of peer attention as the function. Particularly with students in junior high school and above, peer attention and approval become more precious for many students. Hence, conditions in which such is available make the behaviors that recruit such become more likely.

The following factors point to an SMA 2.2 classification: (a) reliable relation between behavior and hypothesized reinforcer (peer attention); (b) behavior seems to be more effective than other behaviors at procuring peer attention; and (c) the MC seems to be a desire for peer attention when it is not currently realized, but is available.

Case 4

Let us postulate that these rude and disrespectful comments that Susan exhibits several times a week serve SME 4.3 Escape from Difficult Tasks/Chores/Assignments.

Question: What would you see happen (what does the classroom staff do) subsequent to Susan saying, "This is stupid!" What would be the antecedent MC?

(Answer on next page)

Case 4

If the function of such rude comments is to terminate the MC for an SME 4.3 category, then staff would mediate such behavior by removing the difficult task or material. The removal of difficult material could be in the form of sending Susan somewhere such as the principal's office, thus terminating the task. But this would also be the case for other functions, particularly SME 4.2: lengthy tasks, chores, or assignments.

The difference would be that such behavior would occur primarily to task difficulty as the MC rather than just tasks of any difficulty level. Given that the curriculum material in most classrooms usually does not vary significantly with respect to grade level across days or weeks, additional testing would be needed to ascertain the putative function. The difficulty of the material as the MC would be established by conducting the divergent validity test for an SME 4.3 (i.e., testing the effect of presenting very easy material). If a differential result occurs between easy and current (difficult) tasks, one can confirm that the removal of tasks is a function of task difficulty, and not simply the presence of any task.[1]

---

1   I believe that this is often referred to as the "can't versus won't" dichotomy.

Case 5

You have been referred a case involving a student, Brian, with severe intellectual disabilities, who pinches staff. Pinching results reliably when he is physically guided to comply with a self-care task (that he cannot do). Such pinching results in the termination of the physical guidance and task 50% of the time. When Brian is physically guided for other tasks that he is capable of doing independently, pinching rarely occurs.

Question: Which of the following three categories is most likely the function: SMA 2.1, DE 3.3 or SME 4.3? Detail the rationale for your answer.

(*Answer on next page*)

Case 5

*Answer:*_____

Since the pinching alters the willingness of the staff to carry out the physical guidance (a reduction of 50% of the opportunities to perform this task), it is a socially mediated escape function. It is not a direct function! A direct function behavior probably occurred in the genesis of the current problem. The student probably learned to ignore staff requests to proceed to the bathroom when it was time for this chore. However, it would have been rendered less effective when staff began guiding Brian to the task. So it would be necessary to respond to the guidance in a manner that makes that intervention less fruitful. But which SME function is most suitable?

The answer lies in the information that the target behavior, pinching, occurs to a task that Brian cannot. In addition, pinching does not occur when guidance is provided for tasks he can do. Hence the paramount MC is one of difficulty of the task or chore; therefore SME 4.3: Difficult Tasks/Chores/Assignments. If it was merely noncompliance to directives or requests, then the more appropriate category would be SME 4.1: Unpleasant Social Situations.

Case 6

Tamika, a 4-year-old preschool student in a special education program, screams when she is told she will have to wait awhile before she can go outside to play.

Question: If screaming is functional, what does it eventually produce via staff mediation of the screaming? What is the MC?

(*Answer on next page*)

Case 6

The MC for Tamika's screaming is the postponing of access to the playground area. In simple terms, Tamika is not able to wait for an indefinite period of time to go play outside. Hence, screaming occurs to the MC for an SMA 2.3 function. Screaming probably has a history of being an effective and efficient manner of getting outside quicker than if she were to just wait. This does not imply that it produces quicker access 100% of the time! It just requires that the release of Tamika to the play area is contingent on screaming some percentage of the time. Simply releasing her in close temporal proximity to the screaming (or at the end of a more lengthy bout) would produce such a function.

Case 7

Suppose that screaming is functional in the previous scenario with Tamika.

Question: What would we know about her pleading with preschool staff to go outside when told she has to wait? Which behavior becomes more probable when she is told to wait? Why?

(*Answer on next page*)

Case 7

*Answer:*_____

If pleading occurred in the past, it was probably ineffective; hence, a lowering of the probability of occurrence to this MC (given its failure to produce the desired outcome). Screaming produced a much better "track record." Hence, Tamika resorts to screaming and not to pleading when there is great desire to go play outside without waiting several minutes to be released. Another important factor may be following "law of child nature." Being among the first students to be released to the outside play area translates to getting on one of the five swings available and not having to wait for someone to get off.

Case 8

Roberto is a special education student who receives his math content in the general education class. Roberto cannot add or subtract, but everyday his assignment in math period involves fourth grade math problems (as specified in the individual education plan [IEP]). The fourth grade teacher wants to discuss the appropriateness of his inclusion program during math as a result of a host of disruptive behaviors that end in Roberto being sent back early to special day class.

Question: What function would appear to be most likely the operable one for the disruptive behaviors in the fourth grade general education class?

(*Answer on next page*)

Case 8

While such a scenario plays out often across many classrooms, the putative function is fairly clear—SME 4.3: Difficult Tasks/Chores/ Assignments. If such is the case, presenting seatwork that is one grade level below his current ability (as a test) should verify such a contention.

The following factors point to this classification: (a) reliable relation between behavior and termination of difficult material (being sent back to special education program would probably result in work that is less of a mismatch); (b) behavior seems to be more effective than other behaviors at being dismissed from general education class (hence socially mediated); and (c) the MC would seem to be the difficulty of the material when compared to the material he receives in special education class.

Case 9

In the case of Roberto, just described, suppose that escape constitutes an SME 4.2.

Question: What would the previously identified function look like (i.e., how would it differ)? What would the data show as far as Roberto's ability to perform the general education class assignments?

(*Answer on next page*)

Case 9

*Answer:*_____

If the target behavior was the result of lengthy task assignments in the mainstream class, two pieces of evidence would be critical to such a contention. First, Roberto would be capable of performing the tasks assigned in the general education class. This could be ascertained by examining standardized test scores in addition to placing a contingency on accuracy and fluency on a probe test day that presents the typical seatwork assignments. For example, the teacher would provide just a small sample of the assignment and designate access to a preferred event immediately after completion (to maximize his motivation to succeed), *if done accurately and fluently.* If Roberto is able to achieve this contingency, it would lend support to a SME 4.2. If the opposite is true—that is, he is unable to perform at mastery levels—then SME 4.3 would be more pertinent for this student's behavioral classification of function.

Second, Roberto would probably show variable daily performance across time in the beginning. On some days he might engage for some time before engaging in disruptive behavior. On other days it might occur much sooner as the instructional session begins. This would occur despite the curriculum not changing in difficulty across time.

Case 10

Bob, a junior high student in a general physical education (PE) class, is reported to have frequent complaints about an upset stomach, as well as other somatic complaints. The result is that he is sent to the nurse's office two to three times per week for the last several weeks. His stay in the nurse's office usually overlaps the PE period. These somatic complaints were reported to surface around the same time period that several boys in the PE class began calling Bob names (in a sly and surreptitious manner, when the PE teacher was busy with other students).

Question: If such an antecedent context is the case, what classification best fits the function of Bob's somatic complaints?

(Answer on next page)

Case 10

The somatic complaints occur in the context of an aversive MC involving "bullying" within a social context. The escape (and probably in some cases, avoidance of such an MC) is the result of teaching staff sending Bob to the nurse's office. The anecdotal report that he often stays there until PE class is over illustrates that this socially mediated function removes his contact with the aversive event: PE class (which has become aversive due to the possibility of bullying incidents).

Case 11

Fred is a 9-year-old child diagnosed with an intellectual disability, but does have the expressive language level of a 4-year-old child. He has been referred for reportedly running out of class once or twice a day. Once he is out of the class, he proceeds to jump on the playground swing and begins playing. The school is required to supervise him at all times; thus a paraprofessional staff person must be outside to ensure his safety without engaging with him. Teaching staff have surmised he does this for their negative attention, and have started ignoring him while he plays on the equipment, unencumbered by staff or other children. This hypothesis leads them to simply wait for him to come in when he sees he is not getting attention.

Question: What would you want to know to discern if such behavior is maintained by attention? What possible direct access function may be at play?

(Answer on next page)

Case 11

This hypothetical case illustrates a common fallacy. As a result of the behavior producing a management and supervision issue, staff members are required to attend to such behavior by being in close proximity to the student when he leaves the classroom. Staff may also admonish him as he heads out the door. They erroneously conclude that this behavior is the result of its ability to recruit staff attention. Hence they have decided to simply wait for him to come back inside, of his own accord. I guess this is the equivalent of teaching-on-demand; whenever Fred is ready to enter the instructional program, teaching will ensue. He seems to be the one in charge of deciding when it is a suitable time.

For attention to be a viable function, one would have to see that other behaviors in Fred's repertoire are not effective at recruiting staff attention. Hence a low rate of such would be existent, especially when compared to other students' access to attention. The divergent validity test would provide such data.

The mistake in this case is not recognizing that such behavior directly contacts the desired tangible reinforcer, playground equipment and solitary play activities. The most suitable diagnostic category is DA 1.2: Tangible Reinforcers. The key information leading to this selected function is the following: (a) reliable relation between behavior and hypothesized reinforcer (outside play activities); (b) behavior seems to be more effective than other behaviors at procuring such; and (c) the MC seems to be a desire for that activity at those times because of its direct relationship with the behavioral chain of leaving the classroom.

APPENDIX A
HYPOTHETICAL EXAMPLES OF TRIGGER ANALYSIS

TRIGGER ANALYSIS FOR DA 1.2: TANGIBLE REINFORCER

Referral: A student leaves a special education preschool classroom unauthorized between one and three times a week, typically in the afternoon.

Presumed function: DA 1.2: Tangible Reinforcer (leaves classroom to play on playground swing after lunch recess period is over).

Contriving the motivating condition (MC): The teacher allows the student to play on the swing at the end of the recess period. After several minutes (at which point such an activity would still be desired), she requests all the students to go back to the classroom. This creates a state of deprivation with respect to this play activity for this particular student. Once inside the classroom, the teacher leaves the student alone in the classroom while everyone transitions to the next activity. By not being in close proximity, the opportunity to engage in the direct access target behavior becomes more readily available. Being less supervised during the initial transition activity following recess has been the context in which such running out of the classroom becomes probable. Other inappropriate behaviors (if they occur), such as requests to go outside or crying, will not result in being allowed outside (since this is a test for a direct access function).

Ceiling limit: The ceiling limit is about 10 minutes, or once the student becomes engaged in the designated classroom activity.

Target problem behaviors: Leaving the classroom unauthorized.

Scoring of trial: If target behavior, leaving the classroom and going to the swings, occurs within the ceiling limit, score a plus; otherwise score a minus for nonoccurrence. The test trial will end when the target behavior occurs. The teacher will be instructed to provide the outside activity for a designated short period of time prior to bringing the student back inside the classroom.

Hypothetical data

Date	Trial	Plus or Minus	Comments
3/16	1	+	
3/17	2	+	
3/20	3	+	
3/21	4	+	
3/22	5	+	

Proportion of trials target behavior occurred: 5/5 (100%).
Proportion of trials target behavior occurred during divergent validity test: 0/5 (0%).

TRIGGER ANALYSIS SMA 2.1: ADULT/STAFF ATTENTION

Referral: A student in a special day class at an elementary school is reported to be impulsive and immature for age (appears that tantrum behaviors are the primary observable problem).

Presumed function: SMA 2.1: Adult/Staff Attention (attention from Ms. Jones, the teacher, when she is busy with someone else).

Contriving the MC: The teacher initially provides attention in close proximity to the student for a short period of time. A state of deprivation for attention is contrived by the teacher subsequently leaving him (i.e., withdraws attention) and attends to another student for up to 8 minutes.

Ceiling limit: 8 minutes.

Target problem behaviors: Tantrums consisting of crying or falling to the floor and crying, or both.

Scoring of trial: If target behavior, crying, occurs within ceiling limit, score a plus; otherwise score a minus for nonoccurrence. The trial will end when the target behavior occurs. The teacher will be instructed to provide attention to the target student at that point.

Hypothetical data

Date	Trial	Plus or Minus	Comments
3/26	1	+	
3/27	2	–	
3/28	3	+	
3/29	4	–	
3/30	5	+	

Proportion of trials target behavior occurred: 3/5 (60%).
Proportion of trials target behavior occurred during divergent validity test: 0/5 (0%).

TRIGGER ANALYSIS SMA 2.3: TANGIBLE REINFORCER

Referral: A student with intellectual disabilities in a middle school special education program has been referred for property destruction.

Presumed function: SMA 2.3: Tangible Reinforcer (makes loud demands and if such are not appeased by allowing him to go outside, he starts throwing items off of nearby tables until he is told to go outside and cool off).

Contriving the MC: The teacher will initially allow the student to play on the swing at the end of the recess period. After several minutes (whereby such an activity would still be desired), she will have Billy and the rest of the class go back to the class. The MC for this activity, that is, swinging on the swings, will be contrived when she brings him back to the classroom (thus removing him from the activity and setting up a state of deprivation with respect to this activity).

Ceiling limit: 10 minutes.

Target problem behaviors: Loud demands to go outside and/or property destruction (throws items off a table).

Scoring of trial: If either of the problem behaviors occurs within the ceiling limit, score a plus; otherwise score a minus for nonoccurrence. The trial will end when a loud demand is made, or if property destruction occurs before demand (not usually the case). The teacher will then immediately provide the outside activity for a designated period of time.

Hypothetical data

Date	Trial	Plus or Minus	Comments
4/16	1	−	
4/17	2	+	
4/22	3	+	
4/23	4	−	
4/28	5	−	

Proportion of trials target behavior occurred: 2/5 (40%).
Proportion of trials target behavior occurred during divergent validity test: 5/5 (100%).[1]

---

[1]   Data suggest SMA 2.1 Adult Attention over SMA 2.3.

TRIGGER ANALYSIS DE 3.1: UNPLEASANT SOCIAL SITUATIONS

Referral: A student in a high school mainstream class is referred for failure to follow classroom rules and work cooperatively with other students.

Presumed function: DE 3.1: Unpleasant Social Situations (when presented with a group activity in classroom, the student leaves the group[2]).

Contriving the MC: The teacher will set up the MC for this student during her engagement in an independent seatwork activity. The teacher will unexpectedly request a transition to a small group work activity at a table and then escort the student to the group. The teacher will then leave the area.

Target problem behaviors: Leaves group unauthorized, either by moving back to seat, wandering around the classroom, or leaving classroom.

Ceiling limit: 5 minutes.

Scoring of trial: If the target behavior, leaving the group and/or classroom, occurs within the ceiling limit, score a plus; otherwise score a minus for nonoccurrence. The trial will end when the target behavior occurs (since escape behavior has already produced the removal). The student will be allowed to return to the independent seatwork assignment.

Hypothetical data

Date	Trial	Plus or Minus	Comments
11/16	1	+	
11/17	2	+	
11/20	3	+	
11/21	4	−	
11/22	5	+	

Proportion of trials target behavior occurred: 4/5 (80%).
Proportion of trials target behavior occurred during divergent validity test: 0/5 (0%).

---

2   Such does not happen during independent seatwork.

TRIGGER ANALYSIS DE 3.2: LENGTHY TASKS, CHORES, OR ASSIGNMENTS

Referral: A student with mild intellectual disabilities is referred for creating disruption to the class during seatwork by running out the door.

Presumed function: DE 3.2: Lengthy Tasks, Chores, or Assignments (imposing lengthy math assignments during seatwork).

Contriving the MC: The teacher will provide lengthy seatwork assignments during math period.[3] If the student finishes the initial assignment, the student will be given another lengthy assignment (imposing the "wacky contingency").

Target problem behaviors: Leaves classroom unauthorized by running out the door and sitting in hallway.

Ceiling limit: Entire math period.

Scoring of trial: If the target behavior, leaving the classroom unauthorized, occurs within ceiling limit, score a plus; otherwise score a minus for nonoccurrence. The trial will end when target behavior occurs (since escape behavior has already produced the removal of the work). The teacher will supervise the student for about 2 minutes outside (but say nothing) and then offer the student an alternate activity to get him to come back to the classroom.

---

3   The material should not be difficult for the student, as a category of either DE 3.3 or SME 4.3 should be ruled out prior to this test (see trigger analysis procedures).

Hypothetical data

Date	Trial	Plus or Minus	Comments
3/16	1	–	
3/17	2	–	
3/20	3	+	
3/21	4	–	
3/22	5	+	Run a few more trials
3/23	6	–	
3/27	7	–	
3/28	8	–	

Proportion of trials target behavior occurred: 2/8 (25%).
Proportion of trials target behavior occurred during divergent validity test: 0/5 (0%).[4]

---

4   Data suggest neither function is operative in this case—suspect SME 3.3 or 4.3 classification if this was not tested first (task difficulty).

TRIGGER ANALYSIS DE 3.3: DIFFICULT TASKS, CHORES, OR ASSIGNMENTS

Referral: A student is referred for not following rules or directives (to come back to class after he has left).

Presumed function: DE 3.3: Difficult Tasks, Chores, or Assignments (imposing difficult math assignments during seatwork).

MC: The teacher will contrive the MC for this student by providing difficult seatwork assignments at the onset of math period.

Target problem behaviors: Leaves classroom unauthorized by running out the door and sitting in hallway.

Ceiling limit: 10 minutes.

Scoring of trial: If the target behavior, leaving the classroom unauthorized, occurs within ceiling limit, score a plus; otherwise score a minus for nonoccurrence. The trial will end when target behavior occurs (since escape behavior has already produced the removal of the work). The teacher will supervise student for about 2 minutes outside and then offer an alternate easier seatwork activity to get the student back in the classroom.

Hypothetical data

Date	Trial	Plus or Minus	Comments
9/6	1	+	
9/7	2	+	
9/8	3	+	
9/9	4	+	
9/13	5	+	

Proportion of trials target behavior occurred: 5/5 (100%).
Proportion of trials target behavior occurred during divergent validity test: 0/5 (0%).

TRIGGER ANALYSIS SME 3.4: AVERSIVE STIMULI

Referral: A referral is made for a student with special needs in junior high school who frequently leaves the physical education (PE) locker room (and sometimes campus), thus creating a supervision problem. He also sometimes fails to bring his gym shorts to school.

Presumed function: SME 3.4: Aversive Stimuli (avoidance of PE class where student is when requested to put on gym shorts).

MC: The PE teacher will contrive the MC by asking this student to dress out for gym period.

Target problem behaviors: Leaves locker area or gym and/or fails to bring gym shorts to school.

Ceiling limit: 10 minutes or subsequent to the student actually putting on gym clothes (rarely happens).

Scoring of trial: If the student begins to leave the locker room area or gym within the ceiling limit, score a plus; otherwise score a minus for nonoccurrence. The trial will end when the student attempts to leave the locker room area. The student will immediately be told that he can go to PE in dress clothes.

Hypothetical data

Date	Trial	Plus or Minus	Comments
9/6	1	+	
9/7	2	+	
9/8	3	+	
9/9	4	+	
9/13	5	+	

Proportion of trials target behavior occurred: 5/5 (100%).
Proportion of trials target behavior occurred during divergent validity test: 0/5 (0%).

TRIGGER ANALYSIS SME 4.1: UNPLEASANT SOCIAL SITUATIONS

Referral: A student in a high school mainstream class is referred for failure to follow classroom rules and work cooperatively with other students.

Presumed function: SME 4.1: Unpleasant Social Situations (when presented with a group activity in classroom, the student makes negative verbal comments, for example, "I don't like working with you! This is stupid!"). Sometimes aggressive behavior occurs following verbal comments, especially when such comments do not result in the student being directed back to seatwork.

Contriving the MC: The teacher will contrive the MC for this student during her engagement in an independent seatwork activity. The teacher will unexpectedly request and then escort the student to transition to a small group work activity at a table. The teacher will then monitor the area.

Target problem behaviors: Negative verbal comments and/or aggressive behavior toward peers.

Ceiling limit: 5 minutes.

Scoring of trial: If negative verbal comments occur within ceiling limit, score a plus; otherwise score a minus for nonoccurrence. The trial will end when the first negative comment occurs (to avoid generating aggressive behavior). The teacher will immediately dismiss the student from the group and return the student to the previous independent seatwork activity.

Hypothetical data

Date	Trial	Plus or Minus	Comments
3/16	1	+	
3/17	2	+	
3/20	3	+	
3/21	4	−	
3/22	5	+	Aggressive behavior occurred first

Proportion of trials target behavior occurred: 4/5 (80%).
Proportion of trials target behavior occurred during divergent validity test: 0/5 (0%).

TRIGGER ANALYSIS SME 4.2: LENGTHY TASKS, CHORES, OR ASSIGNMENTS

Referral: A student with mild intellectual disabilities is referred for creating disruption to class by having severe tantrum episodes.

Presumed function: SME 4.2: Lengthy Tasks, Chores, or Assignments (imposing lengthy math assignments during seatwork).

Contriving the MC: The teacher will contrive the MC for this student by providing lengthy seatwork assignments during math period.[5] If the student finishes the initial assignment, another lengthy assignment is provided (imposing the "wacky contingency").

Target problem behaviors: Tantrum episodes can include any or all of the following: crying, hitting desk, verbally abusive statements such as "I hate you!" and other similar statements, falling on the floor, and kicking the air and/or a close object (e.g., desk).

Ceiling limit: Entire math period.

Scoring of trial: If any form of the target behavior occurs within ceiling limit, score a plus; otherwise score a minus for nonoccurrence. The trial will end when the target behavior occurs. The teacher will immediately offer the student a break from seatwork.

Hypothetical data

Date	Trial	Plus or Minus	Comments
9/6	1	+	
9/7	2	+	
9/8	3	-	
9/9	4	+	
9/13	5	+	

Proportion of trials target behavior occurred: 4/5 (20%).
Proportion of trials target behavior occurred during divergent validity test: 0/5 (0%).

---

5   The material should not be difficult for the student, as a category of either DE 3.3 or SME 4.3 should be ruled out prior to this test (see trigger analysis procedures).

TRIGGER ANALYSIS SME 4.3: DIFFICULT TASKS, CHORES, OR ASSIGNMENTS

Referral: A referral is made for a student in junior high school who has been sent to the principal's office 13 times in the last 2 months for disrespectful behavior.

Presumed function: SME 4.3: Difficult Tasks, Chores, or Assignments (imposing difficult math assignments during seatwork).

MC: The teacher will contrive the MC for this student by providing difficult seatwork assignments at the onset of math period.

Target problem behaviors: Disrespectful behavior can include rude and profane comments to the teacher, subsequent to a directive to initiate work on the assignment.

Ceiling limit: 10 minutes.

Scoring of trial: If the student makes a rude or profane comment to the teacher within the ceiling limit, score a plus; otherwise score a minus for nonoccurrence. The trial will end when the target behavior occurs. The student will subsequently be provided with easier math material (one grade level below his standardized test score). If necessary, the student will be sent to the principal's office with the easier material if the problem behavior creates a significant disruption to the class.

Hypothetical data

Date	Trial	Plus or Minus	Comments
9/6	1	+	
9/7	2	+	
9/8	3	+	
9/9	4	+	
9/13	5	+	

Proportion of trials target behavior occurred: 5/5 (100%).
Proportion of trials target behavior occurred during divergent validity test: 0/5 (0%).

TRIGGER ANALYSIS SME 4.4: AVERSIVE STIMULI

Referral: A referral is made for a student in junior high school who adamantly and profusely refuses to put on gym shorts.

Presumed function: SME 4.4: Aversive Stimuli (engages in severe tantrums when requested to put on gym shorts).

MC: The PE teacher will contrive the MC by asking this student to dress out for gym period.

Target problem behaviors: Tantrum behavior can include loud verbal refusal, lying on floor while screaming, and hitting lockers with fists.

Ceiling limit: 10 minutes.

Scoring of trial: If the student engages in any form of tantrum behavior within the ceiling limit, score a plus; otherwise score a minus for nonoccurrence. The trial will end when the target behavior occurs. The student will subsequently be allowed to leave the locker room and go to PE in dress clothes.

Hypothetical data

Date	Trial	Plus or Minus	Comments
9/6	1	+	
9/7	2	+	
9/8	3	+	
9/9	4	+	
9/13	5	+	

Proportion of trials target behavior occurred: 5/5 (100%).
Proportion of trials target behavior occurred during divergent validity test: 0/5 (0%).

APPENDIX B
REPORT FORMAT[20] FOR FBAs

---

20 This material contained in this appendix can be used in whole for individualized education plans (IEPs) and/or functional behavioral assessment (FBA) reports. Please use proper citation when using classifications categories (Cipani & Cipani, 2017). Also, if a person has behaviors that serve different functions do a separate form for each different function.

Generic Explanation of Function

The specific action of a behavior results in sensory effects (e.g., auditory stimuli, visual stimuli). A specific sensory effect can maintain the explicit form of the action under the motivating condition (state of deprivation with respect to such a reinforcer). The probability of such a form of behavior becomes heightened when there exists a sufficient desire for such a sensory effect.

Specific sensory event believed to be reinforcing:

_____

Specific example(s) of function with individual (specify the behavior that produces putative sensory reinforcer):

_____

Evidence for Selected Function (Chapter 2 methods from Cipani & Schock, 2011):

_____

SELECTED DIAGNOSTIC CLASSIFICATION: DA 1.2: TANGIBLE REINFORCERS *(CIPANI & CIPANI, 2017)*

Generic Explanation of Function

When the absence of an item, activity, or event for a period of time creates a *sufficient* state of deprivation (desire) for this individual, the problem target problem behavior(s) is more likely to occur. The target problem behavior(s) is more effective than other behaviors in accessing the desired item, activity, or event under these motivating conditions (when such is highly valued).

Problem behaviors that produce such a function (under motivating condition):

_____

Specific item(s), activity(ies), and/or event(s) that is desired:

_____

Specific example(s) of function with individual (specify the manner in which attention is obtained):

_____

Evidence for selected function (Chapter 2 methods from Cipani & Schock, 2011):

_____

SELECTED DIAGNOSTIC CLASSIFICATION: SMA 2.1: ADULT ATTENTION *(CIPANI & CIPANI, 2017)*

Generic Explanation of Function

When the absence of adult attention for a period of time creates a *sufficient* state of deprivation (desire) for this individual, the problem target problem behavior(s) is more likely to occur. The target problem behavior(s) is relatively more effective than other behaviors in accessing the desired attention under these motivating conditions (when adult attention is highly valued).

Problem behaviors that produce such a function (under motivating condition):

_____

Specific adult(s) whose attention is desired:

_____

Specific form(s) of attention desired:

_____

Specific example(s) of function with individual (specify the manner in which attention is obtained):

_____

Evidence for selected function (Chapter 2 methods from Cipani & Schock, 2011):

_____

SELECTED DIAGNOSTIC CLASSIFICATION: SMA 2.2: PEER ATTENTION (CIPANI & CIPANI, 2017)

Generic Explanation of Function

When the absence of peer attention or approval for a period of time creates a *sufficient* state of deprivation (desire) for this individual, the problem target problem behavior(s) is more likely to occur. The target problem behavior(s) is relatively more effective than other behaviors in accessing the desired attention under these motivating conditions (when peer attention is highly valued).

Problem behaviors that produce such a function (under motivating condition):

_____

Specific peer(s) whose attention or approval is desired:

_____

Specific form(s) of attention desired:

_____

Specific example(s) of function with individual (specify the manner in which attention is obtained):

_____

Evidence for selected function (Chapter 2 methods from Cipani & Schock, 2011):

_____

Generic Explanation of Function

When the absence of an item, activity, or event for a period of time creates a *sufficient* state of deprivation (desire) for this individual, the problem target problem behavior(s) is more likely to occur. The target problem behavior(s) is more effective than other behaviors in accessing the desired item, activity, or event under these motivating conditions (when such is highly valued). This outcome is achieved by someone providing the item, activity, or event.

Problem behaviors that produce such a function (under motivating condition):

Specific item(s), activity(ies), and/or event(s) that is desired:

Specific example(s) of function with individual (specify the manner in which attention is obtained):

Evidence for selected function (Chapter 2 methods from Cipani & Schock, 2011):

Generic Explanation of Function

When the student is presented with a relatively unpleasant social situation (or impending), thus creating a motivating condition for this individual, the problem target problem behavior(s) is more likely to occur. The target problem behavior(s) is more effective than other behaviors in directly terminating or avoiding such situations. Hence, such a direct form of escape behavior, *for example, leaving the area, situation by oneself,* becomes very probable when the individual wishes to terminate or avoid such situations.

Problem behaviors that produce such a function (under motivating condition):

Specific social situations that create this motivating condition:

Specific example(s) of function with individual (specify the manner in which escape occurs directly from the chain of behaviors that produce such):

Evidence for selected function (Chapter 2 methods from Cipani & Schock, 2011):

SELECTED DIAGNOSTIC CLASSIFICATION: DE 3.2: LENGTHY TASKS, CHORES, OR ASSIGNMENTS *(CIPANI & CIPANI, 2017)*

Generic Explanation of Function

When the student is presented with relatively lengthy tasks, chores, or assignments (or impending), thus creating a motivating condition for this individual, the problem target problem behavior(s) is more likely to occur. Such lengthy instructional conditions usually involve a designated time period for engagement irrespective of the amount of work completed. If the initial assignment is completed, such an outcome brings an additional assignment, until the instructional period elapses. "Finish your work; get more" reflects a "Wacky Contingency."[21] An aversive instructional condition exists because the designated tasks, chores, or assignments continue beyond the individual's current ability to persist in engaging in such instructional task(s).

The target problem behavior(s) is more effective than other behaviors in directly terminating or avoiding such instructional conditions. Hence, such behavior, *for example, leaving the area, desk, task by oneself*, becomes very probable under such motivating conditions (when escaping or avoiding such instructional periods is highly valued).

Problem behaviors that produce such a function (under motivating condition):

_____

Specific tasks, chores, or assignments that create this motivating condition:

_____

Specific example(s) of function with individual (specify the manner in which escape occurs directly from the chain of behaviors that produce such):

_____

Evidence for selected function (Chapter 2 methods from Cipani & Schock, 2011):

_____

---

21   Instead of allowing performance to generate a more preferred activity; hence, completion results in a punishing contingency rather than one of reinforcement (Cipani & Schock, 2011).

SELECTED DIAGNOSTIC CLASSIFICATION: DE 3.3: DIFFICULT TASKS, CHORES, OR ASSIGNMENTS (CIPANI & CIPANI, 2017)

Generic Explanation of Function

When the student is presented with relatively difficult tasks, chores, or assignments (or impending), thus creating a motivating condition for this individual, the problem target problem behavior(s) is more likely to occur. The presentation of such tasks creates an instructional mismatch between the grade level of the content of the curriculum the student must perform daily versus the student's current ability level. The target problem behavior(s) is more effective than other behaviors in terminating or avoiding such tasks. Hence, such behavior, for example, leaving the area, desk, task, or assignment by oneself, becomes very probable under such motivating conditions (when escaping or avoiding such instructional periods is highly valued).

Problem behaviors that produce such a function (under motivating condition):

———————————————————————————————

Specific tasks, chores, or assignments that create this motivating condition:

———————————————————————————————

Specific example(s) of function with individual (specify the manner in which escape occurs directly from the chain of behaviors that produce such):

———————————————————————————————

Evidence for selected function (Chapter 2 methods from Cipani & Schock, 2011):

———————————————————————————————

Generic Explanation of Function:

When relatively aversive stimuli are present (or impending), thus creating a motivating condition for this individual, the problem target problem behavior(s) is more likely to occur. The target problem behavior(s) is more effective than other behaviors in terminating or avoiding aversive physical stimuli. Hence, such behavior, for example, leaving or avoiding the area where such stimuli are present by oneself, becomes very probable (when escaping or avoiding such aversive stimuli is highly valued).

Problem behaviors that produce such a function (under motivating condition):

_____

Specific aversive stimuli/events/items that create this motivating condition:

_____

Specific example(s) of function with individual (specify the manner in which escape occurs directly from the chain of behaviors that produce such):

_____

Evidence for selected function (Chapter 2 methods from Cipani & Schock, 2011):

_____

SELECTED DIAGNOSTIC CLASSIFICATION: SME 4.1: UNPLEASANT SOCIAL SITUATIONS (CIPANI & CIPANI, 2017)

Generic Explanation of Function:

When the student is presented with a (or impending) relatively unpleasant social situation, thus creating a motivating condition for this individual, the problem target problem behavior(s) is more likely to occur. The target problem behavior(s) is more effective than other behaviors in terminating or avoiding such situations than other behaviors. This outcome is achieved by someone producing such a result (i.e., terminating or removing unpleasant social situations). Hence, such behavior becomes very probable when the individual wishes to escape or avoid such situations.

Problem behaviors that produce such a function (under motivating condition):

Specific social situations that create this motivating condition:

Specific example(s) of function with individual (specify the manner in which the behavior achieves escape via social mediation):

Evidence for selected function (Chapter 2 methods from Cipani & Schock, 2011):

SELECTED DIAGNOSTIC CLASSIFICATION: SME 4.2: LENGTHY TASKS, CHORES, OR ASSIGNMENTS *(CIPANI & CIPANI, 2017)*

Generic Explanation of Function:

When the student is presented with relatively lengthy tasks, chores, or assignments (or impending), thus creating a motivating condition for this individual, the problem target problem behavior(s) is more likely to occur. Such lengthy instructional conditions usually involve a designated time period for engagement irrespective of the amount of work completed. If the initial assignment is completed, such an outcome brings an additional assignment, until the instructional period elapses. "Finish your work; get" more reflects a "Wacky Contingency."[22] An aversive instructional condition exists because the designated tasks, chores, or assignments continue beyond the individual's current ability to persist in engaging in such instructional task(s).

The target problem behavior(s) is more effective than other behaviors in directly terminating or avoiding such instructional conditions. This outcome is achieved by someone producing such a result (i.e., terminating or removing task, chore, or assignment). Hence, such behavior becomes very probable under such motivating conditions (when escaping or avoiding such instructional periods is highly valued).

Problem behaviors that produce such a function (under motivating condition):

Specific tasks, chores, or assignments that create this motivating condition:

Specific example(s) of function with individual (specify the manner in which the behavior achieves escape via social mediation):

Evidence for selected function (Chapter 2 methods from Cipani & Schock, 2011):

---

22   Instead of allowing performance to generate a more preferred activity; hence, completion results in a punishing contingency rather than one of reinforcement (Cipani & Schock, 2011).

Generic Explanation of Function

When the student is presented with relatively difficult tasks, chores, or assignments (or impending), thus creating a motivating condition for this individual, the problem target problem behavior(s) is more likely to occur. The presentation of such tasks creates an instructional mismatch between the grade level of content of the curriculum the student must perform daily versus the student's current ability level. The target problem behavior(s) is more effective than other behaviors in terminating or avoiding such tasks than other behaviors. This outcome is achieved by someone producing such a result (i.e., terminating or removing the difficult task). Hence, such behavior becomes very probable under such motivating conditions (when escaping or avoiding such instructional periods is highly valued).

Problem behaviors that produce such a function (under motivating condition):

_____

Specific tasks, chores, or assignments that create this motivating condition:

_____

Specific example(s) of function with individual (specify the manner in which the behavior achieves escape via social mediation):

_____

Evidence for selected function (Chapter 2 methods from Cipani & Schock, 2011):

_____

Generic Explanation of Function

When relatively aversive stimuli are present (or impending), thus creating a motivating condition for this individual, the problem target problem behavior(s) is more likely to occur. The target problem behavior(s) is more effective than other behaviors in terminating or avoiding aversive physical stimuli. This outcome is achieved by someone producing such a result (i.e., terminating or removing aversive stimulus). Hence, such behavior becomes very probable under such motivating conditions (when escaping or avoiding such aversive stimuli is highly valued).

Problem behaviors that produce such a function (under motivating condition):

Specific aversive stimuli/events/items that create this motivating condition:

Specific example(s) of function with individual (specify the manner in which the behavior achieves escape via social mediation):

Evidence for selected function (Chapter 2 methods from Cipani & Schock, 2011):

ALSO OF INTEREST

Functional Behavioral Assessment, Diagnosis, and Treatment:
A Complete System for Education and Mental Health Settings
Ennio Cipani and Keven Schock

Unlike any other book, this text pioneers the authors' unique behavioral classification system for diagnosing the function of problem behaviors, suitable across many different clinical populations. It develops a conceptual understanding of behavioral function, which may not be explored as extensively in other material. Such an understanding is needed to discern which tests or methods are desirable in varied clinical situations! If you are not using this text in your program, talk to a colleague whose program has adopted it; I am confident that you will feel compelled to adopt it for your students. A common anecdote is that "students love the text," in large part due to the plethora of actual and hypothetical examples depicting 13 access and escape functions of The Cipani Behavioral Classification System.

The text also includes the following:

- Extensive instructional resources in electronic form; for example, extensive test bank, lecture slides across all four chapters, instructor overview of text, additional articles, and handouts on direct contingency functions with clinical examples, and more
- Extensive student and faculty ancillary materials that dovetail with book; for example, narrated presentations that interface with text, a study guide tied to each chapter, electronic handouts on differential reinforcement, and more
- Separate chapters on assessment methods for determining the function of behavior and functional treatment
- Recurring hypothetical examples used across different chapters, providing a view of program design across stages of the process
- Multiple treatment options for each type of major function, including *tolerance training option;* and an entire chapter devoted to protocols for each of the major functions, using a hypothetical example that outlines the process from the start of referral to treatment evaluation

The text can be used across several different courses—for example, behavioral functional assessment and intervention/application courses as a secondary adopted text—and is also well suited for practicum courses to structure student activities involving FBAs. The focus on clinical applications makes it relevant in several courses.

If you desire a complete system for teaching students "why" behavior occurs, and "what" to do about it, *this text is a must for your* training program! We believe it is unlike any other text in that regard.

—Ennio Cipani

EXAM COPY AVAILABLE at www.springerpub.com/functional-behavioral-assessment-diagnosis-and-treatment-second-edition.html. Click on supplementary materials link on this page for downloadable narrations that accompany Chapter 1.

REFERENCES

American Psychiatric Association. (2013). Diagnostic and statistical manual of mental disorders (5th ed.). Arlington, VA: American Psychiatric Publishing.

Beavers, G. A., Iwata, B. A., & Lerman, D. C. (2013). Thirty years of research on the functional analysis of problem behavior. *Journal of Applied Behavior Analysis, 46*, 1–21.

Cipani, E. (1990). The communicative function hypothesis: An operant behavior perspective. *Journal of Behavior Therapy and Experimental Psychiatry, 21*, 239–247.

Cipani, E. (1994). Treating children's severe behavior disorders: A behavioral diagnostic system. *Journal of Behavior Therapy and Experimental Psychiatry, 25*, 293–300.

Cipani, E. (2014). Co-morbidity in DSM in childhood mental disorders: A functional perspective. *Research in Social Work Practice, 24*, 78–85.

Cipani, E., & Schock, K. M. (2007). *Functional behavioral assessment, diagnosis, and treatment: A complete system for education and mental health settings* (1st ed.). New York, NY: Springer Publishing.

Cipani, E., & Schock, K. M. (2011). *Functional behavioral assessment, diagnosis, and treatment: A complete system for education and mental health settings* (2nd ed.). New York, NY: Springer Publishing.

Hanley, G. P., Iwata, B. A., & McCord, B. E. (2003). Functional analysis of problem behavior: A review. *Journal of Applied Behavior Analysis, 36*, 147–185.

Michael, J. (1993). Establishing operations. *Behavior Analyst, 16*, 191–206.

Michael, J. L. (2007). Motivating operations. In J. O. Cooper, T. P. Heron, & W. L. Heward (Eds.), *Applied behavior analysis* (2nd ed., pp. 374–391). Upper Saddle River, NJ: Pearson.

Querim, A. C., Iwata, B. A., Roscoe, E. M., Schlichenmeyer, K. J., Ortega, J. V., & Hurl, K. E. (2013). Functional analysis screening for problem behavior maintained by automatic reinforcement. *Journal of Applied Behavior Analysis, 46*, 47–60.

Rolider, A., & Axelrod, S. (2000). *Teaching self-control to children through trigger analysis*. Austin, TX: Pro-Ed.

INDEX